New Insights in Perioperative Care

Edited by Nabil A. Shallik

Published in London, United Kingdom

New Insights in Perioperative Care
http://dx.doi.org/10.5772/intechopen.1001500
Edited by Nabil A. Shallik

Contributors
Adriana Antonucci, Aftab Mohammad Azad, Ahmed Aboelezz, Ahmed Shaban, Alberto Altarocca, Amandeep Virk, Amr Ashour, Baha Hamdi Alkahlout, Belal Khalil, Bruno Carriero, Clemens Kietaibl, Dario Perugia, Dilara Göçmen, Dilar Costa, Domenico Topa, Eman E. Shaban, Fabrizio Marzano, Hany A. Zaki, Hugo de Jesus Ballesteros Loyo, Joana Silva, Jéssica Oliveira, Maria del Carmen Renteria Arellano, Mohamed Hussein, Mustafa Rehan, Nabil A. Shallik, Nicola Filippi, Riccardo Lanzetti, Samuel Davies, Scott Leslie, Sebastiano Porcino, Valerio Pace, Victor Yu, Wenjie Zhong

First published in London, United Kingdom, 2024 by IntechOpen
IntechOpen is the global imprint of INTECHOPEN LIMITED, registered in England and Wales, registration number: 11086078, 167-169 Great Portland Street, London, W1W 5PF, United Kingdom

British Library Cataloguing-in-Publication Data
A catalogue record for this book is available from the British Library

Additional hard and PDF copies can be obtained from orders@intechopen.com

New Insights in Perioperative Care
Edited by Nabil A. Shallik
p. cm.
Print ISBN 978-0-85466-470-2
Online ISBN 978-0-85466-469-6
eBook (PDF) ISBN 978-0-85466-471-9

For EU product safety concerns:
IN TECH d.o.o., Prolaz Marije Krucifikse Kozulić 3, 51000 Rijeka, Croatia,
info@intechopen.com or visit our website at intechopen.com.

Meet the editor

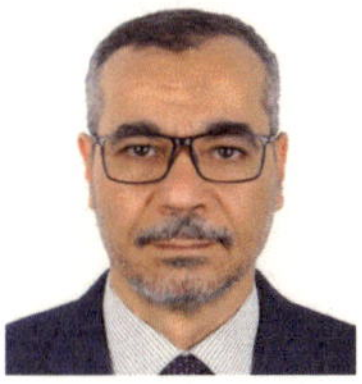

Dr. Nabil A. Shallik, MD, is an associate professor of clinical anesthesiology at Weill Cornell Medical College, Qatar University, Qatar and Tanta University, Egypt. He is the IT deputy chair of the Anaesthesia Department and associate head of anesthesia services in the Ambulatory Care Centre (ACC), Hamad Medical Corporation, Qatar. He also works as a senior consultant for anesthesia, ICU, and perioperative medicine at Hamad General Hospital, Qatar. He has published more than 100 articles in national and international peer-reviewed medical journals, including perioperative, pain, and airway publications. He is also a reviewer and editorial board member for many international peer-reviewed medical journals. He is the principal author of numerous book chapters and editor of many books. He is a leading researcher in airway management in the Middle East, and his research interests focus on perioperative care and new tools for airway assessment and management.

Contents

Preface

Perioperative medicine refers to the medical health care provided to patients preparing for surgery, undergoing surgery, or recovering from surgery. Managing operative risks, complications, and medical diseases are the main aims of perioperative medicine.

For several years, we have felt the necessity for a concise, readable, but comprehensive clinical review book for perioperative medicine. Such a book should be easy to read and provide sound practical advice for both trainees and practitioners.

In combination, knowledge and technology have the immense power to improve healthcare services. This is achieved by the excellent use of the best technology for managing medical diseases and the treatment of patients. This book covers both basic and advanced topics and includes an evidence-based scientific background that is designed to help the user apply theoretical knowledge to actual patient situations.

This volume is intended to be a practical book, not just to be read and placed on a shelf, but hopefully, one that will be taken into the workplace and used as an aid during clinical practice.

While this book is mainly intended for anesthesia trainees and consultants, we believe it would be well suited for intensive care physicians, emergency physicians, surgeons, nurses, anesthesia technical staff, medical students, and pulmonologists.

While we did our best to prevent any misinformation of any form, we would urge our readers to inform us of any errors, including spelling or contextual errors. We also would advise that this book certainly does not replace professional or expert guidance and consultation.

We wish to thank our authors once again for participating in the writing of this important book. We have all benefited from their clinical wisdom and commitment.

I would also like to thank my wife, my sons, and my daughter for their patience and constant support while editing this unique book.

A special thanks to the Department of Anaesthesia, ICU and Perioperative Medicine, Hamad Medical Corporation, and departmental leaders (Drs. Mohamed Hilani and Mashael Al-Khelaifi) for their tireless support, encouragement, and guidance.

Thank you and enjoy your book!

Dr. Nabil A. Shallik
Anaesthesia, ICU and Perioperative Medicine,
Hamad Medical Corporation,
Doha, Qatar

Clinical Anesthesiology,
Weill Cornell Medical College in Qatar,
Doha, Qatar

Clinical Anesthesiology,
Qatar University,
Doha, Qatar

Chapter 1

Enhanced Recovery after Surgery (ERAS) in Hip and Knee Replacement Surgery: Current Concepts and Future Trends

Valerio Pace, Fabrizio Marzano, Bruno Carriero, Nicola Filippi, Adriana Antonucci, Domenico Topa, Sebastiano Porcino, Alberto Altarocca, Dario Perugia and Riccardo Lanzetti

Abstract

Enhanced recovery after surgery (ERAS) protocols have been recently studied and introduced in order to provide and develop peri-operative multidisciplinary programs able to shorten length of hospital stay (LOS), reduce complications, readmissions and costs for patients undergoing major surgery. The number of patients requiring and undergoing total knee replacement and total hip replacement surgery has been increasing for years; however individualized and standardized rehabilitation protocols after surgery are still lacking in most centers. Postoperative joint function, pain control, patient satisfaction, shortest possible length of stay and better quality of life are uppermost priorities for results related to patients undergoing joint replacement surgery. Therefore the knowledge and possibly the implementation of such protocols should be taken into account by all institution. In fact, by utilizing ERAS protocols, the orthopedic surgeons would be able to deliver not just good results strictly related to the surgery itself, but also provide good results in terms of pain, function, mobility, patients' satisfaction, and complications compared to patients undergoing routine rehabilitation. There is enough scientific evidence that ERAS protocols should be seen as a valuable and efficient aid for the orthopedic surgeons and a safe and effective option of the patient after joint arthroplasty surgery.

Keywords: ERAS, joint reconstruction, joint arthroplasty, hip replacement, knee replacement, rehabilitation

1. Introduction

Enhanced recovery after surgery (ERAS) protocols have been initially studied and proposed by the Danish surgeon H. Kehlet in the 1990s. The original idea was to implement a number of measures with regards to perioperative treatments and rehabilitation, basing his research on the scientific evidence available at that time. The final aim was to improve clinical and functional results and accelerate the recovery process together with patient satisfaction and quality of life. Perhaps these goals do not differ much from the ones looked for these days. The good results of ERAS programs have attracted growing acceptance and worldwide adoption [1–3].

ERAS protocols have been successfully proposed and introduced in several specialties and related surgical options. Results have been reported to be good overall in most specialties. ERAS was initially centered on abdominal and colorectal surgery patients but its use was then extended to many other specialties, including orthopedic surgery (mainly total hip and knee replacement surgery) [1, 2]. The focus of our chapter is on ERAS protocols for hip or knee replacement surgery and therefore we will keep our attention strictly on these areas.

The basic principles of ERAS protocols are shared among researchers and clinicians: using the least invasive surgical practices; reducing complications; reducing costs; reducing length of stay at hospitals; improving patients' satisfaction and postoperative quality of life; fastest possible recovery; better clinical and functional outcomes; better postoperative pain control. Good results have been achieved due to substantial improvements in the fields of orthopedic surgical techniques and anesthetic management strategies. With regards to costs, it must be said that a huge burden is linked to the postoperative care after joint replacement surgery. In fact, a relevant amount of money is spent on physical and occupational therapy, nutrition and social services [1–3].

The combination of interventions included in these protocols are thought to reduce the post-op surgical stress response and overall optimize the perioperative wellbeing of the patients undergoing hip and knee arthroplasty surgery. In fact, major orthopedic surgeries are naturally followed by a pathophysiologic catabolism e slow recovery and the proposed interventions must overcome these adverse factors [1, 4].

Recent high level of evidence research reported that the measures used to analyze the outcomes have initially been related to costs, length of stay, readmission rates and complication rates. More recently further attention has been given to more subjective outcome measures, such as patient reported outcome measures (PROMs) which include satisfaction and quality of life (QoL) scores, meaning that the patient experience is these days considered as important as clinical related aspects as indicators of quality. In some countries (e.g. United Kingdom, United States) PROMs are standardly recorded for patients undergoing elective hip and knee replacement procedures [4, 5]. The use of national joint registries have certainly helped researchers and clinicians in carrying out relevant research on this topic [6].

It has been well reported that the demographic changes in the last few decades (significant and progressive age of the populations) make us predict that total primary hip replacements (THR) and total knee replacements (TKR) will keep increasing in numbers. Patients do not just evaluate results strictly related to the surgical procedures but their dissatisfaction could be related to chronic pain or limitation of function postoperatively [5, 6]. Therefore these two aspects must be particularly looked after when performing such type of surgery and a multidisciplinary approach and interventions seem to be the perfect strategy in order to obtain the best possible objective and subjective outcomes [1, 5, 6].

Despite a huge number of studies have been published on ERAS programs (some of which with high level of evidence), it has been reported overall inconsistent data availability on the efficacy and reproducibility of ERAS protocols and their real impact on early postoperative pain. The most recent literature reviews reveals a certain amount of uncertainty and show the need for further research and meta-analysis on this field in order to uniformly utilize and access these programs and create share-standardized knowledge among orthopedic surgeons around the world [1, 2, 5, 6].

Our aim was to provide all the relevant up to date information on ERAS protocols in relation to hip and knee replacement surgery, highlighting the most current known aspects and concepts, the weaknesses, potential room for improvement, the available most recent scientific evidence and suggesting future research directions and trends.

A literature review was performed using the following search database: Pubmed, Embase and Cochrane. Relevant key words were searched: "ERAS", "Enhanced Recovery After Surgery", "ERAS Orthopedic", "ERAS knee surgery", "ERAS hip surgery", "ERAS joint arthroplasty", "ERAS joint replacement", "ERAS hip replacement", "ERAS knee replacement". All articles were scrutinized and 40 papers were finally included.

2. Enhanced recovery after surgery (ERAS) in hip and knee replacement surgery

Enhanced recovery after surgery (ERAS) protocols in joint arthroplasty surgery are programs based on scientific evidence aimed to deliver a standardized, multimodal and multidisciplinary perioperative management which should provide a quicker and more efficient recovery after surgery as well as the best possible clinical and functional outcomes. This approach should indirectly guarantee reduced complication rates, shorter length of stay, better patient satisfaction. In simple words these protocols are built to target the main factors that could delay the postoperative recovery [1–7].

Many articles with different level of evidence have been published over the last few decades, proposing internationally standardized ERAS programs. However, at the same time, many institutions have developed their own individualized programs after considering their own specific financial burden and particular types of surgery. With regards to orthopedic surgery, there is clear evidence that ERAS programs improve both hospital and patient outcomes [7, 8].

The studied ERAS interventions for primary THR and TKR that have been reported (in different combinations) are as follows: least invasive surgical approach, spinal anesthesia, intraoperative and postoperative local infiltration analgesia, femoral blocks, patients' education before undergoing surgery (related to pain management, gait training such as walking with crutches and specific exercises), pre-op non-steroid-anti-inflammatory-drugs, intravenous application of a steroid, patient-controlled analgesia, continuous femoral nerve block, tranexamic acid intravenously as well as topically or intra-articularly, no use of wound drains, first mobilization 2–4 hours after surgery, intensive physiotherapy by special trained therapists, immediate full weight bearing allowed, adequate analgesia, nutrition support for specific conditions (such as anti-anemic or hypoproteinemia therapy, postoperative nutrition supplement, ice therapy [1, 4–6].

The relevant outcomes measures reported in different combinations in ERAS protocols are: length of incision, length of stay, operation time, intraoperative blood loss, pre and post-op hemoglobin, pre and post-op albumin, costs, readmission rates, complications rates, patient reported outcome measures (PROMs), range of motion (ROM), numerical Rating Scale (NRS), Lysholm score, Oxford Knee Score (OKS), wound delayed healing, surgical site infection, use of pre and post-op opioids, Harris Hip Score, Oxford Hip Score [1, 4–6].

The common interventions used in orthopedic ERAS programs have been divided into those performed in the preoperative, intraoperative, and postoperative phases of care [7–10].

2.1 Pre-operative phase

Several systematic reviews have reported that preoperative patient education could be beneficial for patients undergoing orthopedic surgery as it could reduce preoperative anxiety. However, his positive effects on independently improving the postoperative outcomes is doubtful. These findings have been however described by not sufficiently powered studies and therefore the need for further randomized controlled studies has been advocated. Certainly preoperative education could not be harmful and could provide good support and counseling for the patients. Preoperative education may represent a useful adjunct, with low risk of undesirable effects, particularly in certain patients, for example people with depression, anxiety or unrealistic expectations, who may respond well to preoperative education that is stratified according to their physical, psychological and social need [9, 10].

The multidisciplinary team delivering an ERAS program should take into account the preoperative risk factors that could lead to delayed recovery or, even worse, complications. All specific individual factors should be identified and analyzed. This is supported by the ERAS evidence-based literature [8, 10].

Smoking has been found as a factor able to increase the length of stay, postoperative mortality and complication rate. ERAS protocols should include a smoke cessation program, to be started at least 4 weeks before surgery. The evidence related to these aspects is level 1 and 2 [10–13]. Similar findings were highlighted with regards to alcohol consumption. Again, studies showed that patients who misused alcohol had increased complication rates and longer length of stay. Therefore, an alcohol cessation intervention is recommended before orthopedic surgery [9, 14].

Another aspect to be considered preoperatively is the hematic levels of hemoglobin and hematocrit. It has been shown that anemia could cause an increased risk of transfusion, length of stay, infection, morbidity, and readmission rates. To battle this issue, some ERAS protocols have included the use of preoperative iron or erythropoietin therapy and postoperative re-transfusion of salvaged cells. The cause of the anemia must also be investigated and managed [9, 15, 16].

Despite the current evidence does not fully support the use of carbohydrate loading, few studies have reported its benefits in the perioperative period as it could potentially reduce the preoperative hunger and nausea and the postoperative pain and glucose metabolism. However, it is clear that further studies are needed in order to provide high level of evidence [9, 17, 18].

Differently, there is strong evidence on the timing of intake of clear fluids (until 2 hours before the anesthesia induction) and solid food (up to 6 hours before the anesthesia induction). Factors such as timing of surgery with regards to the operating list and individual aspects should be considered by the anesthetist [9, 19].

Preoperative physiotherapy has been widely and commonly considered very important for patients undergoing joint replacement surgery. However, there is little evidence that it could expedite recovery and discharge. It seems that preoperative physiotherapy could particularly help patients in the first post-op days, whilst his efficacy on the medium and long term is doubtful [9, 20, 21].

Pre-existing conditions such as coronary artery disease, hypertension, chronic obstructive pulmonary disease, diabetes and organ dysfunction are strong determining factors of postoperative complications and duration of hospital stay. It is crucial to meet with patients several weeks before their scheduled surgery. It allows the preoperative team to optimize any organ dysfunction, address issues that may cause any potential risk, and to optimize preoperative anemia. It also gives the opportunity to initiate alcohol and smoking cessation programs if indicated (**Table 1**) [7, 22].

2.2 Peri-operative phase

Most of the aspects related to this phase are anesthesia related. There are minimal data supporting the use of sedative or anxiolytic drugs used before the anesthesia takes places. Even if their use could help the patient to feel more comfortable and less stressed in proximity of the anesthetic and surgical procedure, they could cause side effects such as sedation [23].

Standardized anesthetic protocols should be used and integrated in ERAS protocols. Most of recent high level of evidence studies have favored the use of neuraxial anesthesia over general anesthesia. In fact, relevant literature fully support neuraxial anesthesia and its advantages in terms of reduced complications and better results [9, 24, 25].

Despite the adjunct of opioids to local anesthetic in spinal anesthesia could cause an increased risk of urinary retention and respiratory depression, a low opioids dose could lower these risks and at the same time reinforce the effect of the anesthetic on pain. However, their use is still debated, as the related side effects are relatively common and potentially very dangerous [9, 26].

ERAS interventions		
Preoperative	**Intra-perioperative**	**Postoperative**
Patient education	Sedative or anxiolytic drugs	To manage nausea and vomiting
Preoperative risk factors	Neuraxial anesthesia	Multimodal analgesia approach
Smoking cessation	Opioids in spinal anesthesia	PCA and as required opioids
Avoid alcohol consumption	Local infiltration analgesia or nerve blocks	Antibiotic/antiseptic prophylaxis
Hematic levels of hemoglobin	Venous thromboembolism prophylaxis	Venous thromboembolism prophylaxis
Carbohydrate loading	Minimally invasive surgical technique	Early mobilization
Timing of intake of clear fluids	Maintaining normothermia through forced air warming	Tailored rehab approach to patients
Preoperative physiotherapy	Optimal intraoperative fluid balance	No use of tourniquet
Considerations of pre-existing conditions	Blood conservation	No use of drains
	Intravenous or infiltrative tranexamic acid	No urinary catheter when possible
		Postoperative nutritional care

Table 1.
Preoperatively, intra-perioperative and postoperative ERAS interventions.

The use of local infiltration analgesia or nerve blocks is still debated. It is unclear whether one technique is superior over the other. Moreover, there are studies reporting similar results with a postoperative wound infusion catheter technique, as long as multimodal, oral non-opioid analgesia [26, 27]. There are several nerve block techniques that may be used. Some studies have reported good results with femoral nerve blockade, which is probably the most used technique for total knee replacements. The Hunter Canal block is an alternative to the femoral nerve block and is proposed to offer better preserved quadriceps muscle strength and mobilization ability in the 48 hours post-surgery. Differently, no significant advantages have been proved to be given by sciatic nerve blocks [9, 26–29].

The opoioid crisis seen worldwide has prompted a multimodal approach to pain management in the preoperative, perioperative, and postoperative periods. For example, NSAIDs, acetaminophen, preoperative bupivicane, adenosine, magnesium, clonidine, and venlafaxine have all been effective analgesics in patients undergoing orthopedic surgery (and other types of surgery too). There is also evidence that sedatives and anxiolytics can be avoided with appropriate preoperative counseling, whereas histamine H2 blockers and proton pump inhibitor prophylaxis can be used in patients who have had a shortened fasting period [7, 9].

There is evidence suggesting that regional anesthesia confers a greater advantage in total joint arthroplasty from a physiological standpoint. It is sufficient for surgery, provides a sympathetic block, inhibits stress hormone release, and decreases insulin resistance. Reduced length of stay is also associated with the use of neuraxial anesthesia as opposed to general anesthesia. Epidurals in major open surgeries have been shown to decrease respiratory complications and decrease bowel ileus as opposed to general anesthesia with concurrent opioid use. Many ERAS protocols advocate a multimodal approach to pain management to limit opioid use. Additionally, neuraxial techniques have been shown to blunt the stress response and decrease length of stay, which are all important in extended recovery programs [7, 9, 30].

Aspects related to venous thromboembolism (VTE) prophylaxis characterized both the pre, peri and postoperative phase. Unfractionated and low molecular weight heparin is the most common prophylaxis strategy used internationally. Surgical societies all over the world have follow their own recommendations. VTE prophylaxis is usually recommended for at least 14 days post-op. Most of societies recommend against the use of VTE prophylaxis 12 hours prior to insertion or removal of a catheter (**Table 1**) [7, 30].

2.3 Intra-operative phase

The general aim of the multidisciplinary ERAS team during the intra-operative phase is to reduce the physical stress of the surgery. The trauma-induced physiological responses should be kept under controlled and reduced to the lesser possible level. As mentioned in the previous section, neuraxial anesthesia has always been preferred and considered superior to general anesthesia in ERAS protocols. Local infiltration analgesia (LIA) is administered by surgeons intraoperatively, in and around the joint. Ropivacaine is most commonly used as local anesthetic, mixed with epinephrine and/or steroids. LIA is more useful when used in total knee arthroplasty. It provides postoperative pain relief 6–12 h after total knee arthroplasty. However, when used in total hip arthroplasty, it has no analgesic effect [7, 31].

The orthopedic surgeons themselves obviously play an important role in this "game". The most minimally invasive surgical technique should be planned and performed by the surgeons. Major orthopedic surgery does not often allow room for small surgical wounds, but a big effort should be made in order to use the least invasive approach and protect relevant anatomical structures throughout the entire procedure. This is thought to reduce the physical stress of the surgery, complications, wound healing and pain levels [1, 2, 7, 9].

Other precautions that should attract the attention of the surgical and anesthetic team are: maintaining normothermia through forced air warming (this is associated with reduced infections, coagulopathy, blood transfusion rate, and cardiovascular complications, mainly because of reduced cortisol and catecholamine release; several associations recommends the pre-warming of patients and to maintain the active warming of all adults undergoing surgery throughout the intraoperative phase); optimal intraoperative fluid balance (this assures a better tissue oxygenation and a quicker wound healing process); blood conservation strategies (preoperative anemia should be investigated and corrected through the use of iron supplements or erythropoietin; blood salvage techniques should be utilized in surgical theaters, allowing a reduced need for allogeneic transfusions; the use of intravenously or infiltrative tranexamic acid, an antithrombotic drug able to reduce blood loss and the need for blood transfusions) (**Table 1**) [7, 9, 30, 32].

2.4 Post-operative phase

Postoperative nausea and vomiting can cause significant discomfort to patients in the first days after surgery and determining prolonged length of stay and delayed rehabilitation progress. Therefore, the use of dopamine antagonists, serotonin antagoinists and corticosteroids (or a combination of these) should be taken into account by the multidisciplinary team.

A multimodal analgesia approach (mainly non-opioid oral analgesia) is recommended and advocated. In fact, a combination of different analgesics classes together with the use of different modes of action is associated with better pain control and reduced need for the use of opioids. Paracetamol and non-steroidal anti-inflammatory drugs (NSAIDs) are the mainstay. Optimal pain management is a prerequisite of ERAS and alternative analgesic drugs (such as glucocorticoids, gabapentinoids and ketamine) have been described for hip and knee replacement. In the postoperative phase, several combination of epidural analgesia, continuous or patient-controlled, peripheral nerve blocks, single injection or continuous, acetaminophen, NSAIDs, gabapentin, and ketamine, have all been used for the same purpose [7, 9, 33, 34].

The use of opioids should be limited but their used has been reported in some centers using ERAS protocols, despite their well-known potential side effects. They are often used with a "as required" modality in the very few hours/days after surgery. Different opioids have been studied, among which oxycodone and sulfentanil. Initially a PCA (patient controlled analgesia) regime could be initiated, to be then switched to oral medications [7, 9, 35].

There is currently no universal internationally defined guideline for antibiotic/antiseptic prophylaxis for hip and knee replacement, with differing national and local policies in existence. However, a recent consensus paper does present recommendations for type, timing, dosing, and repetition of antimicrobials [36, 37].

Deep venous thrombosis (DVT) and pulmonary embolism (PE) are two of the most common and impactful complications following THR and TKR surgery. Again, there is no universal international consensus with regards to type and timing of prophylaxis. A minimum of 14 days of antithrombotic prophylaxis (up to 4–5 weeks) is usually recommended. Early mobilization and a tailored approach are certainly the new trends in this field, but further evidence is needed in order to validate the current research [1, 2, 7, 9].

Other aspects that should attract the attention of the surgical and anesthetic team are: the use of tourniquet for TKR surgery (many recent studies discourage its use as it could increase the risk of wound complications, DVT and slower functional recovery); the use of drains (recent studies have shown no advantages with its use as their use could cause increased risk of wound infections, hematomas and wound healing complications); the use of indwelling urinary catheters (despite being routinely utilized, recent high level of evidence studies reported increased incidence of renal and urological complications against no evidence of benefits by the use of urinary catheters); postoperative nutritional care (early return to normal diet is encouraged in most of ERAS protocols, despite the absence of high level of evidence) [7, 9, 35, 38, 39].

A mainstay of ERAS protocols is certainly early mobilization following surgery. Patients should be mobilized as soon as possible following surgery. It has been well studied and proved that prolonged bed rest postoperatively is associated with increased risk of thromboembolism, pulmonary complications, insulin resistance, and delayed wound healing. There are centers reporting patients' discharge within 48–72 hours after surgery, with the support of studies with level 1 evidence. A well trained and specialized team of physiotherapists are necessary in order to achieve such good results, in the few hours/days after surgery as well as in the following weeks. A preoperative assessment to identify the patient's expectations and the goals of rehabilitation and a tailored approach in the postoperative phase are the keys for the best possible results (**Table 1**) [7, 9].

3. Discussion and conclusions

ERAS protocols are a combination of interventions based on the most scientific evidence and characterized by a tailored approach for each patient. This approach was initially hypothesized and introduced in abdominal surgery, and then adopted in orthopedic surgery for elective hip and knee arthroplasty [1–9].

The use of ERAS programs has demonstrated to provide excellent results with regards to both clinical-functional outcomes and the subjective patient experience before, during and after joint arthroplasty surgery. The most relevant positive aspects of ERAS protocols related to orthopedic surgery studied and recorded are: using the least invasive surgical practices; reducing complications; reducing costs; reducing length of stay at hospitals; improving patients' satisfaction and postoperative quality of life; fastest possible recovery; better clinical and functional outcomes; better postoperative pain control [1–4, 7–9].

The ERAS pathway consists of a selected number of interventions divided into those performed preoperatively, intraoperatively, and postoperatively (**Table 1**). All of them play a relevant and complementary role for the common aim to achieve the best possible objective and subjective outcome [7, 9].

Despite their great success and high level of evidence from a scientific point of view, ERAS programs are not routinely used and their widespread use is far from being achieved. Researchers attribute the responsibility for the latter issue to several factors: not satisfactory surgical team education and patients' education; difficulties in changing the traditional practice; potential costs of ERAS implementations (education, rehabilitation centers, equipment, size of the team looking after patients, etc.…). One could argue that these issues could be counterbalanced, point by point, by the improvements that could be achieved through the use of ERAS implementations. Despite any positive considerations, ERAS protocols are adapted in very few specialized orthopedic centers around the globe [1, 2, 4, 7, 9].

This chapter summarizes the available evidence and the current knowledge and implementations of ERAS programs for patients undergoing elective THR and TKR. It is evident that a very early discharge (1–3 days) is possible and safe for such patients if ERAS protocols are put in place. Several studies have proposed a number of implementations in relation to ERAS programs: this chapter has widely considered all of them and outlined a useful summary to be utilized by the clinicians dealing with this cohort of patients, after having carefully considered the level of evidence of such studies and not included low level of evidence results.

Our aim is to explain in the most simple and clear way how ERAS programs works and highlight their potential advantages compared to more traditional practice. This should work as a starting point for the clinicians working with THR and TKR patients and as a trigger for reflection on the current practice, in order to find room for improvements. A more broad application (worldwide) of the ERAS implementations could generate further data and evidence, with the final result of better understanding, more standardization and wide international consensus. There are areas that particularly need further research more than the others, such as how to reduce pain and improve function, specific aspects of the post-op inflammatory response, specific aspects related to patients' morbidity (chronic disease, psychiatric disorders, etc.…) [1, 2, 7, 9, 15, 23].

We believe that ERAS in joint replacement surgery is safe and cost effective, and its use should be widely promoted [1, 2, 7, 9, 40]. His use could be applicable to both younger and older patients as research shows its efficacy in providing good clinical-functional results, quicker recovery, low morbidity, low complications rates, shorter length of stay, quick return to independency in the daily activities and better experience for the patients [1–10, 40].

Future research is needed in order to achieve better standardization and high level of evidence for all aspects related to ERAS, including patient experience and subjective results. In fact, the quality of existing evidence is limited due to several aspect, among which heterogeneity of the studies and significant risk of bias. Moreover, further progress should be specifically made in the application of ERAS protocols in THR and TKR surgery, to highlight specific considerations and improvements related to this cohort of patients and the performed surgery.

4. Take home messages

- The number of patients requiring and undergoing total knee replacement and total hip replacement surgery has been increasing for years; however individualized and standardized rehabilitation protocols after surgery are still lacking in most Orthopedic centers.

- Enhanced recovery after surgery (ERAS) protocols have been recently studied and wildly introduced in order to provide and develop peri-operative multidisciplinary programs able to shorten length of hospital stay (LOS), reduce complications, readmissions and costs for patients undergoing major surgery. The knowledge and possibly the implementation of such protocols should be taken into account by all institutions.

- The use of ERAS protocols in hip and knee replacement surgery can allow good clinical-functional results, better pain control, quicker recovery, low morbidity, low complications rates, shorter length of stay, quick return to independency in the daily activities and better experience for the patients with better patient satisfaction.

- There is enough scientific evidence that ERAS protocols should be seen as a valuable and efficient aid for the orthopedic surgeons and a safe and effective option of the patient after joint arthroplasty surgery.

- We believe that ERAS in joint replacement surgery is safe and cost effective, and its use should be widely promoted

- Future research is needed in order to achieve better standardization and high level of evidence for all aspects related to ERAS.

Conflict of interest

The authors declare no conflict of interest.

Appendices and nomenclature

ERAS	enhanced recovery after surgery
LOS	length of stay
PROMSs	patient reported outcome measures
THR	total hip replacements
TKR	total knee replacement
ROM	range of motion
NRS	numerical Rating Scale
OKS	Oxford Knee Score
VTE	venous thromboembolism
NSAIDs	non-steroidal anti-inflammatory drugs
PCA	patient controlled analgesia
DVT	Deep venous thrombosis
PE	pulmonary embolism

Author details

Valerio Pace[1*], Fabrizio Marzano[2], Bruno Carriero[3], Nicola Filippi[4], Adriana Antonucci[5], Domenico Topa[5], Sebastiano Porcino[5], Alberto Altarocca[6], Dario Perugia[7] and Riccardo Lanzetti[5]

1 Trauma and Orthopaedics Department, "AOSP Terni" Hospital, Terni, Italy

2 Trauma and Orthopaedics Department, "Ospedale degli Infermi" Hospital, Faenza, RA, Italy

3 Trauma and Orthopaedics Department, University of Perugia, Perugia, Italy

4 Trauma and Department, U.O.D. Knee Surgery, ASL Viterbo, Viterbo, Italy

5 Orthopaedics and Traumatology Unit, "San Camillo-Forlanini" Hospital, Rome, Italy

6 U.O.C. Spinal Unit and Rehabilitation, Ostia, Rome, Italy

7 Hand Surgery Unit, Orthopaedics and Traumatology Department, University "La Sapienza", Rome, Italy

*Address all correspondence to: valeriopace@doctors.org.uk

References

[1] Zhu S, Qian W, Jiang C, Ye C, Chen X. Enhanced recovery after surgery for hip and knee arthroplasty: A systematic review and meta-analysis. Postgraduate Medical Journal. 2017;**93**(1106):736-742. DOI: 10.1136/postgradmedj-2017-134991

[2] Frassanito L, Vergari A, Nestorini R, Cerulli G, Placella G, Pace V, et al. Enhanced recovery after surgery (ERAS) in hip and knee replacement surgery: Description of a multidisciplinary program to improve management of the patients undergoing major orthopedic surgery. Musculoskeletal Surgery. 2020;**104**(1):87-92. DOI: 10.1007/s12306-019-00603-4

[3] Hernández-Romero CH, Martínez-Montiel O, Blanco-Bucio P, Villalobos-Campuzano CA. Valencia-Martínez G. Impacto del programa "Enhanced Recovery After Surgery" en artroplastía de rodilla a nivel institucional [Impact of the "Enhanced Recovery After Surgery" program in knee arthroplasty at the institutional level]. Acta Ortop Mex. 2023;**37**(1):14-18

[4] Jones EL, Wainwright TW, Foster JD, Smith JR, Middleton RG, Francis NK. A systematic review of patient reported outcomes and patient experience in enhanced recovery after orthopaedic surgery. Annals of the Royal College of Surgeons of England. 2014;**96**(2):89-94. DOI: 10.1308/003588414X13824511649571

[5] Reinhard J, Schindler M, Leiss F, Greimel F, Grifka J, Benditz A. No clinically significant difference in postoperative pain and side effects comparing conventional and enhanced recovery total hip arthroplasty with early mobilization. Archives of Orthopaedic and Trauma Surgery. 2023;**143**(10):6069-6076. DOI: 10.1007/s00402-023-04858-2

[6] Li J, Zhao F, Gao J, Dong W, Yu X, Zhu C, et al. Enhanced recovery after surgery (ERAS) protocol in geriatric patients underwent unicompartmental knee arthroplasty: A retrospective cohort study. Medicine (Baltimore). 2023;**102**(6):e32941. DOI: 10.1097/MD.0000000000032941

[7] Kaye AD, Urman RD, Cornett EM, Hart BM, Chami A, Gayle JA, et al. Enhanced recovery pathways in orthopedic surgery. Journal of Anaesthesiology Clinical Pharmacology. 2019;**35**(Suppl. 1):S35-S39. DOI: 10.4103/joacp.JOACP_35_18

[8] Miller TE, Thacker JK, White WD, Mantyh C, Migaly J, Jin J, et al. Reduced length of hospital stay in colorectal surgery after implementation of an enhanced recovery protocol. Anesthesia and Analgesia. 2014;**118**(5):1052-1061. DOI: 10.1213/ANE.0000000000000206

[9] Wainwright TW, Gill M, McDonald DA, Middleton RG, Reed M, Sahota O, et al. Consensus statement for perioperative care in total hip replacement and total knee replacement surgery: Enhanced Recovery After Surgery (ERAS®) Society recommendations. Acta Orthopedics. 2020;**91**(1):3-19. DOI: 10.1080/17453674.2019.1683790

[10] McDonald S, Page MJ, Beringer K, Wasiak J, Sprowson A. Preoperative education for hip or knee replacement. Cochrane Database of Systematic Reviews. 2014;**2014**(5):CD003526. DOI: 10.1002/14651858. CD003526.pub3

[11] Hansen TB, Bredtoft HK, Larsen K. Preoperative physical optimization in fast-track hip and knee arthroplasty. Danish Medical Journal. 2012;**59**(2):A4381

[12] Singh JA. Smoking and outcomes after knee and hip arthroplasty: A systematic review. The Journal of Rheumatology. 2011;**38**(9):1824-1834. DOI: 10.3899/jrheum.101221

[13] Mak JC, Fransen M, Jennings M, March L, Mittal R, Harris IA. National Health and Medical Research Council (NHMRC) of Australia. Evidence-based review for patients undergoing elective hip and knee replacement. ANZ Journal of Surgery. 2014;**84**(1-2):17-24. DOI: 10.1111/ans.12109

[14] Best MJ, Buller LT, Gosthe RG, Klika AK, Barsoum WK. Alcohol misuse is an independent risk factor for poorer postoperative outcomes following primary Total hip and Total knee arthroplasty. The Journal of Arthroplasty. 2015;**30**(8):1293-1298. DOI: 10.1016/j.arth.2015.02.028

[15] Kehlet H. Fast-track hip and knee arthroplasty. Lancet. 2013;**381**(9878):1600-1602. DOI: 10.1016/S0140-6736(13)61003-X

[16] MuñozM, Gómez-RamírezS, CuencaJ, García-Erce JA, Iglesias-Aparicio D, Haman-Alcober S, et al. Very-short-term perioperative intravenous iron administration and postoperative outcome in major orthopedic surgery: A pooled analysis of observational data from 2547 patients. Transfusion. 2014;**54**(2):289-299. DOI: 10.1111/trf.12195

[17] Soop M, Nygren J, Thorell A, Weidenhielm L, Lundberg M, Hammarqvist F, et al. Preoperative oral carbohydrate treatment attenuates endogenous glucose release 3 days after surgery. Clinical Nutrition. 2004;**23**(4):733-741. DOI: 10.1016/j.clnu.2003.12.007

[18] Awad S, Varadhan KK, Ljungqvist O, Lobo DN. A meta-analysis of randomised controlled trials on preoperative oral carbohydrate treatment in elective surgery. Clinical Nutrition. 2013;**32**(1):34-44. DOI: 10.1016/j.clnu.2012.10.011

[19] Smith I, Kranke P, Murat I, Smith A, O'Sullivan G, Søreide E, et al. Perioperative fasting in adults and children: Guidelines from the European Society of Anaesthesiology. European Journal of Anaesthesiology. 2011;**28**(8):556-569. DOI: 10.1097/EJA.0b013e3283495ba1

[20] Carli F, Zavorsky GS. Optimizing functional exercise capacity in the elderly surgical population. Current Opinion in Clinical Nutrition and Metabolic Care. 2005;**8**(1):23-32. DOI: 10.1097/00075197-200501000-00005

[21] Wang L, Lee M, Zhang Z, Moodie J, Cheng D, Martin J. Does preoperative rehabilitation for patients planning to undergo joint replacement surgery improve outcomes? A systematic review and meta-analysis of randomised controlled trials. BMJ Open. 2016;**6**(2):e009857. DOI: 10.1136/bmjopen-2015-009857

[22] McLeod RS, Aarts MA, Chung F, Eskicioglu C, Forbes SS, Conn LG, et al. Development of an enhanced recovery after surgery guideline and implementation strategy based on the knowledge-to-action cycle. Annals of Surgery. 2015;**262**(6):1016-1025. DOI: 10.1097/SLA.0000000000001067

[23] Møiniche S, Kehlet H, Dahl JB. A qualitative and quantitative systematic review of preemptive analgesia for

postoperative pain relief: The role of timing of analgesia. Anesthesiology. 2002;**96**(3):725-741. DOI: 10.1097/00000542-200203000-00032

[24] McDonald DA, Siegmeth R, Deakin AH, Kinninmonth AW, Scott NB. An enhanced recovery programme for primary total knee arthroplasty in the United Kingdom--follow up at one year. The Knee. 2012;**19**(5):525-529. DOI: 10.1016/j.knee.2011.07.012

[25] Khan SK, Malviya A, Muller SD, Carluke I, Partington PF, Emmerson KP, et al. Reduced short-term complications and mortality following Enhanced Recovery primary hip and knee arthroplasty: results from 6,000 consecutive procedures. Acta Orthopedics. 2014;**85**(1):26-31. DOI: 10.3109/17453674.2013.874925

[26] Andersen LØ, Kehlet H. Analgesic efficacy of local infiltration analgesia in hip and knee arthroplasty: A systematic review. British Journal of Anaesthesia. 2014;**113**(3):360-374. DOI: 10.1093/bja/aeu155

[27] McCartney CJ, McLeod GA. Local infiltration analgesia for total knee arthroplasty. British Journal of Anaesthesia. 2011;**107**(4):487-489. DOI: 10.1093/bja/aer255

[28] Jaeger P, Nielsen ZJ, Henningsen MH, Hilsted KL, Mathiesen O, Dahl JB. Adductor canal block versus femoral nerve block and quadriceps strength: A randomized, double-blind, placebo-controlled, crossover study in healthy volunteers. Anesthesiology. 2013;**118**(2):409-415. DOI: 10.1097/ALN.0b013e318279fa0b

[29] Paul JE, Arya A, Hurlburt L, Cheng J, Thabane L, Tidy A, et al. Femoral nerve block improves analgesia outcomes after total knee arthroplasty: A meta-analysis of randomized controlled trials. Anesthesiology. 2010;**113**(5):1144-1162. DOI: 10.1097/ALN.0b013e3181f4b18

[30] Temple-Oberle C, Shea-Budgell MA, Tan M, Semple JL, Schrag C, Barreto M, et al. Consensus review of optimal perioperative Care in Breast Reconstruction: Enhanced recovery after surgery (ERAS) society recommendations. Plastic and Reconstructive Surgery. 2017;**139**(5):1056e-1071e. DOI: 10.1097/PRS.0000000000003242

[31] Alvarez A, Goudra BG, Singh PM. Enhanced recovery after bariatric surgery. Current Opinion in Anaesthesiology. 2017;**30**(1):133-139. DOI: 10.1097/ACO.0000000000000404

[32] Sambandam B, Batra S, Gupta R, Agrawal N. Blood conservation strategies in orthopedic surgeries: A review. Journal of Clinical Orthopedics Trauma. 2013;**4**(4):164-170. DOI: 10.1016/j.jcot.2013.11.002

[33] Ong CK, Seymour RA, Lirk P, Merry AF. Combining paracetamol (acetaminophen) with nonsteroidal antiinflammatory drugs: A qualitative systematic review of analgesic efficacy for acute postoperative pain. Anesthesia and Analgesia. 2010;**110**(4):1170-1179. DOI: 10.1213/ANE.0b013e3181cf9281

[34] Mathiesen O, Jacobsen LS, Holm HE, Randall S, Adamiec-Malmstroem L, Graungaard BK, et al. Pregabalin and dexamethasone for postoperative pain control: A randomized controlled study in hip arthroplasty. British Journal of Anaesthesia. 2008;**101**(4):535-541. DOI: 10.1093/bja/aen215

[35] Husted H. Fast-track hip and knee arthroplasty: Clinical and organizational

aspects. Acta Orthopaedica. Supplementum. 2012;**83**(346):1-39. DOI: 10.3109/17453674.2012.700593

[36] Voigt J, Mosier M, Darouiche R. Systematic review and meta-analysis of randomized controlled trials of antibiotics and antiseptics for preventing infection in people receiving primary total hip and knee prostheses. Antimicrobial Agents Chemotherapy. 2015;**59**(11):6696-6707. DOI: 10.1128/AAC.01331-15

[37] Aboltins CA, Berdal JE, Casas F, Corona PS, Cuellar D, Ferrari MC, et al. Hip and knee section, prevention, antimicrobials (systemic): Proceedings of international consensus on Orthopedic infections. The Journal of Arthroplasty. 2019;**34**(2S):S279-S288. DOI: 10.1016/j.arth.2018.09.012

[38] Prasad N, Padmanabhan V, Mullaji A. Blood loss in total knee arthroplasty: An analysis of risk factors. International Orthopaedics. 2007;**31**(1):39-44. DOI: 10.1007/s00264-006-0096-9

[39] Bjerregaard LS, Hornum U, Troldborg C, Bogoe S, Bagi P, Kehlet H. Postoperative urinary catheterization thresholds of 500 versus 800 ml after fast-track Total hip and knee arthroplasty: A randomized, open-label, controlled trial. Anesthesiology. 2016;**124**(6):1256-1264. DOI: 10.1097/ALN.0000000000001112

[40] Xu S, Liow MHL, Liu XE, Pang HN, Chia SL, Tay KJD, et al. Enhanced recovery after day surgery total knee arthroplasty, the new standard of care: An Asian perspective. The Knee. 2023;**44**:158-164. DOI: 10.1016/j.knee.2023.08.003

Chapter 2

Perioperative Fluid Management

Dilara Göçmen

Abstract

Perioperative fluid management is a critical aspect of surgical care, containing the preoperative, intraoperative, and postoperative phases. Management of patients without individualisation, utilizing established standard protocols, may lead to undesirable events such as hypovolaemia and hypervolaemia during both intraoperative and postoperative periods. Insufficient fluid administration can result in peripheral vasoconstriction, leading to decreased oxygen delivery, impaired tissue perfusion, and dysfunction of vital peripheral organs. Conversely, excessive fluid administration may cause increased vascular permeability due to glycocalyx damage, tissue oedema, impaired tissue perfusion, local inflammation, delayed wound healing, wound infection, and anastomotic leaks. The pursuit of an optimal fluid regimen that prevents volume overload while maximizing tissue perfusion has led to the adoption of individualized, targeted fluid replacement therapies, supported by advancing technology. In this approach, basic physiological variables related to cardiac output or global oxygen distribution are measured. In optimized fluid management, fluid replacement is adjusted according to targeted physiological variables in a continuously re-evaluated process. These physiological variables can be assessed using different methods, from simple tests to complex devices that evaluate the patient's tissue perfusion and cardiac output. Developments in recent years have drawn attention to the future of non-invasive or less invasive cardiac output measurement devices, as well as the utilization of ultrasonographic cardiac output measurements.

Keywords: goal-directed therapy, fluid therapy, hemodynamic monitoring, perioperative care, cardiac output

1. Introduction

Perioperative fluid management is a critical aspect of surgical care, which contains the preoperative, intraoperative, and postoperative phases.

Fluid therapy is essential for treating surgical patients, and it can be lifesaving. Insufficient fluid volume (hypovolemia) can lead to poor circulation, reducing oxygen delivery to organs and peripheral tissues, resulting in organ dysfunction and shock. Conversely, excessive fluid (fluid overload) can cause interstitial oedema, local inflammation, and hinder collagen regeneration, weakening tissue healing and increasing the risk of postoperative complications such as wound infections, wound

IntechOpen

rupture, and anastomotic leakage. Additionally, fluid overload can impair cardiopulmonary function. Therefore, administering fluid therapy on an individual basis, as needed, and in appropriate amounts is essential [1–5].

Perioperative fluid management strategies can be examined in three sections.

2. Preoperative fluid optimization

The body's adaptive mechanisms in hypovolaemia attempt to maintain blood flow to critical organs such as the heart and brain. Peripheral vasoconstriction that develops through this mechanism may have harmful effects on organ function in the perioperative period. This can lead to ischemia in surgical tissues, which require adequate blood flow for tissue repair and healing.

Several factors contribute to reduced effective circulating blood volume in surgical patients. These include preoperative fasting, hypertonic bowel preparations, anesthetic agents, and positive pressure ventilation. Consequently, anesthetized patients often present with a functional intravascular volume deficit [1].

Preoperative hydration is an essential consideration for patient preparation. Studies demonstrate the benefits of preoperative oral carbohydrate solutions over traditional fasting rules, as well as the importance of personalized fluid plans tailored to the patient's needs.

A meta-analysis of existing trials found that a shorter preoperative fasting period did not increase the risk of aspiration or result in larger volumes of gastric content [2].

The current guidelines in Europe and America suggest that clear fluids can be consumed up to 2 hours before elective surgery. A study has demonstrated that correcting intravascular volume deficits before surgery effectively reduces postoperative nausea and vomiting (PONV) as well as postoperative pain in high-risk patients [3].

A large retrospective review found that preoperative dehydration is linked to higher rates of postoperative acute renal failure (ARF), myocardial infarction (MI), and cardiac arrest. Additionally, hydrotherapy for dehydrated patients has been shown to decrease postoperative complications in colorectal surgery [4].

These approaches aim to prevent dehydration and maintain optimal physiological reserves before surgery, contributing to the acceleration of recovery and the reduction of perioperative complications. Individual treatments should be applied to the patient, and both hypovolemia and hypervolemia should be avoided. The main goal should be optimal tissue oxygenation and euvolemia.

3. Intraoperative fluid strategies

Calculating the fluid volume to administer per unit time based on a formula involving body weight, type of surgical trauma, and operation time is not supported by established physiological principles [5]. Studies have indicated that a strategy focusing on hemodynamic stabilization can reduce complications after major surgery [6]. Meta-analyses and reviews have further highlighted the effectiveness of this approach across different patient populations and types of surgeries [6, 7].

A patient's physiological state and hemodynamic stability are complex. The main goals of the applied treatments, including fluid therapy and use of vasoactive drugs such as vasopressors, vasodilators, and inotropes, are to maintain adequate blood volume, perfusion pressure, cardiac output, tissue blood supply, and oxygen delivery.

Fluid therapy is often the first choice for hemodynamic support due to the decrease in circulating blood volume associated with anesthesia and surgery. However, its impact is indirect. Optimizing oxygen delivery and removing metabolic by-products may require a combination of fluid therapy, drugs, and mechanical support.

Both hypovolemia and hypervolemia increase postoperative morbidity. Hypovolemia can cause vasoconstriction, decreased oxygen delivery, reduced tissue perfusion, and dysfunction in peripheral organs. Conversely, hypervolemia can lead to tissue oedema, which can result in worsened tissue perfusion, pulmonary oedema, local inflammation, delayed wound healing, wound site infections, and anastomotic leaks [8]. Intestinal oedema, associated with hypervolemia, is known to increase bacterial translocation and the risk of multiple organ failure syndrome.

Hypervolemia can harm glycocalyx, an endovascular structure vital for endothelial integrity. This damage leads to fluid shifting into the interstitial space. Atrial natriuretic peptide (ANP) is also involved in this process and is secreted during hypervolemia [9]. When the glycocalyx is damaged, as in cases of ischemia, inflammation, surgery, or acute hypervolemia, colloids, and crystalloids leak from the vascular barrier into the interstitial space, resulting in tissue oedema [9, 10].

Fluid infusions directly increase vascular volume, improving perfusion and blood pressure, especially if the heart is responsive. However, these effects depend on the cardiac and peripheral vascular status, leading to varying effects. Therefore, blind fluid infusion or using vasopressors without understanding the patient's cardiovascular status is not advised.

According to the Frank-Starling curve, there is a positive correlation between preload and stroke volume, and this relationship follows a curvilinear shape. A larger increase in stroke volume is observed for a given increase in preload in the steeply rising portion of the curve. This part can be considered as the preload-dependent area. The plateau portion of the curve can be defined as a preload-independent area where volume expansion will not create significant changes in stroke volume. Since left ventricular function reaches its maximum level near the plateau of the Frank-Starling curve, subsequent fluid load has little effect on cardiac output and only causes increased tissue oedema and tissue hypoxia. In daily practice, clinicians evaluate several hemodynamic variables to indicate whether the patient lies in the preload-dependent or preload-independent area of the Frank-Starling curve.

In the operating room, fluid management becomes a dynamic process, requiring careful consideration of fluid types and volumes. Balanced crystalloid solutions remain a cornerstone, but colloids may be indicated in specific cases such as major hemorrhage or hypoalbuminemia. The concept of goal-directed fluid therapy, guided by hemodynamic monitoring, allows for precise fluid administration, minimizing the risk of fluid overload or inadequate perfusion during surgery.

3.1 Goal-directed fluid therapy (GDFT)

The pursuit of an optimal fluid regimen that prevents volume overload while maximizing tissue perfusion has led to the adoption of individualized, targeted fluid replacement therapies, supported by advancing technology. In this approach, basic physiological variables related to cardiac output or global oxygen distribution are measured. The administration of crystalloids, colloids, blood products, or inotropic agents is then dynamically adjusted based on these targeted physiological variables.

Tissue and organ perfusion rely on both perfusion pressure and cardiac output (CO). It is crucial to accurately measure CO, or at least detect changes in CO. While invasive monitoring with a pulmonary artery catheter (PAC) was once the gold standard, many alternative and less invasive devices are now available. The term "Minimally Invasive CO Monitoring" encompasses all devices capable of calculating CO without requiring a PAC. Cardiac output monitor, used alongside protocols to optimize CO and oxygen delivery (DO_2), as well as direct intravenous fluid therapy and inotropic support, are fundamental to targeted fluid therapy. Studies have demonstrated that targeted fluid therapy, when combined with minimally invasive CO monitors, enhances perioperative outcomes in high-risk surgical patients [11].

The objective of intraoperative fluid management is to maintain central euvolemia. Therefore, it is recommended that patients undergoing surgery under the ERAS (Enhanced Recovery After Surgery) protocol have an individualized fluid management plan. Excessive crystalloid use should be avoided in all patients. A "zero balance" approach is encouraged for some patients undergoing low-risk surgery. Goal-directed fluid therapy (GDFT) is recommended for most patients undergoing surgeries involving large fluid shifts. Optimal perioperative fluid management is a critical component of the ERAS protocol. One study demonstrated that simply modifying fluid management on the day of surgery reduced perioperative complications by 50% [8].

Randomized controlled studies and meta-analyses have shown that GDFT reduces postoperative renal damage, postoperative complications, postoperative hospital stay, and mortality [12–15]. Perioperative targeted fluid management algorithms have been shown to be beneficial in high-risk geriatric patients and may reduce the length of hospital stay [16].

Several dynamic parameters are used in GDFT to assess fluid responsiveness and guide fluid administration. By incorporating these dynamic parameters into fluid resuscitation protocols, clinicians can tailor fluid therapy to the individual patient's needs, optimizing hemodynamic status and improving outcomes.

3.1.1 Dynamic methods in determining cardiac preload

Dynamic methods for assessing cardiac preload involve using physiological parameters that change in response to alterations in intrathoracic pressure or volume status. Dynamic parameters provide real-time information about the heart's ability to respond to volume changes, which can help guide fluid therapy in critically ill patients or during surgery.

3.1.1.1 Pulse contour analysis

This is based on the principle that the area under the systolic portion of the arterial pressure waveform is proportional to the stroke volume (SV). It was first described by Erlanger and Hooker in 1904, who suggested that cardiac output (CO) was proportional to arterial pulse pressure [17]. In this method, the area under the curve is measured until the end of the post-diastolic ejection phase and divided by the aortic impedance measuring left ventricular (LV) function. It also measures stroke volume variation (SVV) and pulse pressure variation (PPV), which are useful in estimating fluid responsiveness.

3.1.1.1.1 Pulse pressure variation (PPV)

This dynamic parameter was established by demonstrating changes in stroke volume induced by positive pressure ventilation. Heart-lung interactions during mechanical ventilation and changes in hemodynamic signals with respiration have gained great popularity in recent years [18]. Arterial pulse pressure is calculated as the difference between systolic and diastolic blood pressure. PPV is calculated by dividing the peak pulse pressure (PP) (PPmax – PPmin) by the average PP [(PPmax + PPmin)/2] [19]. Arterial pulse pressure is directly proportional to stroke volume and inversely proportional to the compliance of large systemic arteries. Arterial compliance is assumed to remain constant throughout the respiratory cycle. Therefore, PPV should reflect the magnitude of respiratory-induced changes in stroke volume. Consequently, PPV should predict the degree of biventricular preload response and hence the hemodynamic response to fluid infusion. In conditions where there is no obstacle to the use of this parameter in the patient, if PPV is high and decreases with fluid infusion, the patient can be considered fluid-responsive [18]. Mechanically ventilated patients with normal tidal volume have been the subject of numerous studies in a variety of clinical settings (sepsis, intra-perioperative periods) and these studies have confirmed the excellent value of PPV in predicting fluid response in patients without spontaneous respiratory activity and cardiac arrhythmia [20, 21].

Most studies have also highlighted the clinical utility of PPV, showing that it is much better at predicting fluid response than static preload markers such as cardiac filling pressures. The threshold value of PPV varies between 10% and 15%. Hemodynamic monitors such as PiCCO, VolumeView, LiDCO, MostCare, and Pulsioflex allow automatic calculation of PPV and continuous display on their screens in real time. Therefore, PPV may be a helpful tool to guide volume expansion during surgery as a study done during perioperative phase demonstrated that its capacity to detect a change in cardiac output following volume expansion is better than changes in arterial pressure [22]. As a result, PPV can be used to track the hemodynamic response to fluid therapy in addition to predicting fluid response. to predict fluid response but also to monitor hemodynamic response to fluid therapy. The use of PPV for intraoperative GDFT has been shown to reduce the duration of mechanical ventilation, postoperative complications, and intensive care unit or hospital stay in patients undergoing high-risk surgery [23].

3.1.1.1.2 Stroke volume variation (SVV)

SVV is measured with continuous cardiac output monitoring devices such as FloTrac/Vigileo, PiCCO, LiDCO, MostCare, or esophageal Doppler. It is calculated by dividing the difference between maximum SV and minimum SV (SVmax – SVmin) by their average [(SVmax + SVmin)/2] over a 30-second time window [19]. SVV has been reported as a good predictor of fluid responsiveness in neurosurgical patients, general surgery patients, septic shock patients, and after cardiac surgery [24–27]. In a study conducted on patients who underwent surgery for liver transplantation, a sensitivity and specificity of 94% and a threshold value of SVV of 10% were reported [28]. It has been shown that gastrointestinal complications are reduced in patients undergoing major abdominal surgery who undergo intraoperative SVV-guided GDFT [29].

3.1.1.2 Limitations of pulse contour analysis methods

The most significant limitation is the presence of spontaneous respiratory activity. In a patient with spontaneous respiratory effort, ventilation cannot be provided at regular intervals and with an equal volume of tidal volume. Accordingly, changes in intrathoracic pressure become irregular, and changes in stroke volume are not preload-dependent. The existence of cardiac arrhythmias is another restriction on the use of respiratory variability measures. In these situations, diastolic irregularity rather than heart-lung interactions is responsible for the variation in stroke volume. The final drawback is that the arterial pressure changes brought on by mechanical breathing are likewise minimal in patients with low tidal volume ventilation. Even in reaction to preload, there may not be a sufficient intrathoracic pressure change during low tidal volume breathing. For this reason, studies indicate that PPV is reliable when ventilation is provided with a tidal volume of at least 8 ml/kg [30, 31].

In cases of low lung compliance, changes in alveolar pressure are less effectively transmitted to intrathoracic structures. Consequently, intravascular pressure changes induced by mechanical ventilation may also be diminished. A clinical study demonstrated that PPV loses its ability to predict fluid responsiveness in patients with respiratory compliance less than 30 ml/cm/H_2O [32].

Another limitation is the patient's high respiratory frequency. It has been reported that the reliability of SVV decreases if the ratio of heart rate to respiratory rate is lower than 3.6 or if the respiratory rate exceeds 40/min [33].

It is emphasized that operating room conditions are generally ideal for accurate interpretation of PPV and other respiratory variability indices. Its use has decreased in the intensive care environment where these limitations are common; alternative methods have been developed to estimate fluid response in critically ill patients [18].

1. *End-expiratory occlusion test (EEOT):* EEOT is a preload-dependent method that utilizes heart-lung interactions to estimate fluid response in ventilated patients. It can be used in patients with cardiac arrhythmia or spontaneous ventilator triggering, where parameters like PPV and SVV are not reliable. During a 15-second end-expiratory occlusion (EEO), a greater than 5% increase in arterial pulse pressure measured by the PiCCO device, or in the cardiac index derived from the pulse curve, provides a good prediction of fluid responsiveness [34]. This test is advantageous due to its simplicity. It is considered more reliable than PPV and SVV in patients with acute respiratory distress syndrome (ARDS) characterized by low tidal volume and low lung compliance [32, 35]. However, it cannot be used in patients in whom spontaneous triggering of the ventilator interrupts EEO and, of course, in patients who are not ventilated. Due to its brief duration, EEOT requires the use of a real-time hemodynamic monitor to assess hemodynamic response. Therefore, pulse contour analysis monitors or ultrasound techniques may be appropriate.

2. *Mini fluid challenge test:* Classic liquid loading typically involves infusing 300–500 ml of fluid [36], but its irreversibility can lead to fluid overload, especially with repeated daily administration. To reduce this risk, a 'mini' fluid challenge has been proposed, consisting of a rapid infusion of 100 ml over 1 minute. In clinical studies, an increase of more than 10% in the subaortic velocity time integral, measured using echocardiography, has been found to predict fluid

responsiveness accurately [37]. However, a major limitation of this test is that even in cases of preload responsiveness, a very small volume infusion causes only minimal changes in cardiac output. Therefore, accurate measurement of cardiac output is crucial to minimize false-negative results.

3. *Passive leg raise test (PLRT):* PLRT is independent of heart-lung interactions when assessing preload. Therefore, it can be used in spontaneously breathing patients [38]. Raising the legs from the horizontal position induces a gravitational blood transfer from the lower extremities toward the intrathoracic area. This significantly increases right and left cardiac preload, allowing assessment of the position on the Frank-Starling curve of increased preload during testing [39]. PLRT remains a good indicator of fluid response in patients with acute circulatory failure, spontaneous respiratory activity, or cardiac arrhythmias [40, 41].

   A 10–12% increase in cardiac output or stroke volume during PLRT allows us to predict fluid responsiveness even in patients with cardiac arrhythmias and/or spontaneous ventilator triggering. However, since changes in arterial pressure may result in false-negative cases, cardiac output response should be monitored with real-time cardiac output monitoring technologies and devices to evaluate the hemodynamic response to PLR [38, 42].

   The complete reversibility of PLRT's effects when the legs are returned to the supine position confirms its role as a safe, risk-free preload response test [38, 42]. However, despite its reliability and convenience, PLRT has limitations. It cannot be used in situations where patient mobilization is impossible or prohibited, such as in the operating room or in cases of head trauma [43]. Additionally, the reliability of PLRT is compromised in cases of increased intra-abdominal pressure [44].

4. *Inferior vena cava collapsibility index (cIVC):* The inferior vena cava (IVC) is a low-pressure and highly collapsible vein. Its diameter varies depending on intravascular volume status, right heart function, and respiration [45]. In each respiratory cycle, the IVC contracts and relaxes according to venous return, which changes due to negative pressure. Negative pressure during inspiration increases venous return to the heart, causing the IVC to collapse [46]. Conversely, during expiration, the IVC diameter increases again and returns to its baseline value. These changes in vessel diameter provide guidance in assessing the patient's clinical status.

   In mechanically ventilated patients, the effect of respiration on intrathoracic pressure is completely reversed. Positive pressure applied during inspiration causes venous return to the heart to decrease and the diameter of the IVC to increase. The change in diameter on the IVC in mechanically ventilated patients can be calculated using the 'distensibility index' [47].

   It is believed that the collapse of the IVC during inspiration in spontaneously ventilated patients or the stretching of the IVC during inspiration in mechanically ventilated patients predicts fluid response [48].

IVC ultrasound has several advantages over other fluid response assessment methods. It is non-invasive, inexpensive, widely available, can be obtained with minimal training, can be performed quickly, can be combined with heart and lung ultrasound, and can be repeated frequently [47].

IVC ultrasound is performed with a low-frequency (2–5 MHz) convex probe using the subxiphoid view. The IVC should be viewed longitudinally in the long axis, keeping the connection between the IVC and the right atrium on the screen. The M-mode line should be placed perpendicular to the IVC and 2–3 cm before entering the right atrium. It should be measured at the widest (IVCd-max) and narrowest (IVCd-min) points by monitoring for 2 or 3 respiratory cycles [48].

cIVC is calculated according to the formula:

$$\text{cIVC} = (\text{IVCd-max} - \text{IVCd-min}) / \text{IVCd-max} \times 100 \tag{1}$$

A cIVC value between 40% and 48% could predict fluid response with good specificity and sensitivity, according to studies assessing the usefulness of cIVC as an indicator of fluid response and a guide for fluid management in critically ill patients with acute circulatory failure and spontaneous breathing [31, 46, 49]. Given the circumstances, it seems that very high or very low cIVC values could be helpful in accurately indicating or ruling out fluid responsiveness, particularly in individuals suffering from acute circulatory failure brought on by sepsis. To guide fluid management, cIVC should be interpreted cautiously and considered in conjunction with other parameters, not as a stand-alone parameter [50].

In spontaneously breathing patients undergoing elective non-cardiac surgery, cIVC-directed intravascular fluid therapy before spinal anesthesia has been shown to be an effective method to prevent hypotension after spinal anesthesia [51].

In spontaneously breathing patients, IVC measurements estimate right atrial pressure (RAP), allowing rapid identification of hypovolemic patients [52, 53]. The American Society of Echocardiography states that in measurements with more than 50% collapsed IVC diameter (IVCd) less than 2.1 cm by incision, the right atrial pressure (RAP) is 3 mm Hg (0–5 mm Hg); it is stated that RAP is 15 mm Hg (10–20 mm Hg) in measurements with less than 50% collapse with inspiration and IVCd greater than 2.1 cm [54].

4. Postoperative fluid balance

Following surgery, patients face challenges related to fluid shifts, postoperative stress response, and potential complications such as dehydration or fluid overload. Postoperative patients with extensive traumatic or surgical tissue injury, prolonged surgeries and associated stress response, burns, critical illness, or sepsis require more complex resuscitative fluid therapy in addition to maintenance therapy.

The stress response to traumatic or surgical tissue damage is the "Fight or Flight" response designed to facilitate survival after a major injury. This stress response can occur when the integrity of large body cavities such as the chest, abdomen, joints, and skull is disrupted due to surgery or trauma. It can also be seen in cases of significant tissue damage such as burns, pancreatitis, and gunshot wounds. It may occur in postoperative patients in cases of significant blood loss, hemodynamic instability, and sepsis.

Vasopressin, aldosterone, catecholamines, cortisol, and inflammatory cytokines are secreted in response to stress. These substances affect the patient through various mechanisms, including hemodynamic response, cardiac output, glucose metabolism, and vascular permeability. These effects may occur more intensely in the postoperative period, and fluid management of the patient remains as important as in the intraoperative period.

Individualized postoperative fluid management, coupled with early mobilization, becomes crucial in restoring fluid balance and promoting recovery. Strategies focusing on personalized fluid replacement and monitoring contribute to better postoperative outcomes and reduced recovery times.

1. *Assessment*: assess the patient's fluid status based on clinical signs, urine output, laboratory values (e.g., electrolytes, creatinine), and the type of surgery performed.

   Intravenous fluid administration will not improve tissue perfusion unless it increases stroke volume and, consequently, cardiac output.

   Studies show that almost half of unstable patients do not respond hemodynamically to fluid resuscitation [21, 55]. This indicates that fluid resuscitation may not always be the appropriate approach to ensure adequate tissue perfusion, especially in unstable patients. Therefore, assessing the patient's response to fluid resuscitation should determine the need for additional volume.

2. *Maintenance fluids*: once the patient is stable, maintenance fluids should be provided to replace ongoing losses. The choice of fluids and rate of administration depends on the patient's fluid status, comorbidities, and surgical considerations.

   There are generally two main types of fluids used during major surgery, and the choice of fluid can impact outcomes. The more commonly used type is crystalloid solutions, which remain the fluid of choice for simple postoperative fluid replacement. Crystalloid solutions increase intravascular volume, but their intravascular residence time is shorter than colloids. Prolonged administration of chloride-rich solutions can lead to hyperchloremic acidosis, kidney injury [56–62].

   Compared to crystalloid therapy, colloids require less volume to achieve the same hemodynamic effect. Therefore, the use of colloids can be considered an approach to limit total volumes and could potentially lead to better results. Studies comparing the results of surgical patients receiving colloid or crystalloid fluid replacement generally found no difference [63, 64]. A subgroup analysis of the postoperative population of a large, randomized trial in the intensive care unit found no difference in mortality between crystalloid and colloid-treated populations Although starch solutions can be used intraoperatively, they are not commonly used for volume expansion in postoperative surgical patients due to their potential to cause bleeding or abnormal clotting [65].

3. *Avoiding overhydration*: large volumes of intravenous fluid may cause complications due to the formation of tissue oedema. Liberal administration of fluid may impair pulmonary, cardiac, gastrointestinal, and renal function, contributing to postoperative complications and prolonged recovery [66–69].

4. *Electrolyte monitoring*: monitor electrolyte levels regularly, especially in patients at risk of electrolyte imbalances (e.g., those with renal dysfunction or certain surgical procedures).

   Serum lactic acid, base deficiency, and central venous oxygen saturation (SvO2) are biochemical markers of perfusion frequently used to confirm the adequacy of end-organ perfusion in critically ill patients [70].

5. *Considerations for specific surgeries*: certain surgeries may require special considerations for fluid management. For example, patients undergoing major abdominal surgery may require different fluid strategies than those undergoing minor procedures, extensive traumatic or surgical tissue injury, burns, critical illness, or sepsis require more complex resuscitative fluid therapy.

6. *Individualized approach*: fluid management should be individualized based on the patient's clinical condition, comorbidities, and surgical requirements. Collaborate with the surgical team and other healthcare providers to optimize fluid therapy.

7. *Early mobilization and oral intake*: encourage early mobilization and oral intake as tolerated, as this can help prevent fluid retention and promote recovery.

   Early mobilization is a key element of ERAS protocols for all postoperative patients capable of ambulation [71]. It is essential for reducing the risk of postoperative pneumonia and venous thromboembolism and hospital length of stay.

8. *Monitoring and documentation*: monitor the patient's fluid status closely and document intake, output, and any fluid-related interventions to ensure continuity of care.

9. *Multimodal approach*: consider multimodal approaches to fluid management, including goal-directed therapy and dynamic methods in determining fluid response to optimize outcomes and minimize complications.

5. Future directions

In the future, the integration of emerging technologies and personalized approaches is poised to revolutionize perioperative fluid management. From advanced hemodynamic monitoring to individualized fluid optimization algorithms, the future holds promise for more precise and tailored strategies, ultimately enhancing patient safety and surgical outcomes. Areas for further research include the impact of fluid management on specific patient populations and the development of comprehensive perioperative fluid management guidelines.

6. Conclusion

In conclusion, perioperative fluid management stands as a cornerstone of surgical care, with far-reaching implications for patient recovery and outcomes. By embracing evidence-based practices, individualized approaches, and emerging technologies, healthcare providers can continue to refine perioperative fluid management, paving the way for safer surgeries and improved patient experiences.

Author details

Dilara Göçmen
Department of Anaesthesiology and Reanimation, Marmara University Pendik Training and Research Hospital, Istanbul, Turkey

*Address all correspondence to: dilaragocmen@yahoo.com

References

[1] Bundgaard-Nielsen M, Jørgensen CC, Secher NH, Kehlet H. Functional intravascular volume deficit in patients before surgery. Acta Anaesthesiologica Scandinavica. 2010;**54**(4):464-469. Available from: https://pubmed.ncbi.nlm.nih.gov/20002360/

[2] Brady MC, Kinn S, Stuart P, Ness V. Preoperative fasting for adults to prevent perioperative complications. Cochrane Database of Systematic Reviews. 2003;**2010**(4). Available from: https://pubmed.ncbi.nlm.nih.gov/14584013/

[3] Maharaj CH, Kallam SR, Malik A, Hassett P, Grady D, Laffey JG. Preoperative intravenous fluid therapy decreases postoperative nausea and pain in high risk patients. Anesthesia and Analgesia. 2005;**100**(3):675-682. Available from: https://pubmed.ncbi.nlm.nih.gov/15728051/

[4] Moghadamyeghaneh Z, Phelan MJ, Carmichael JC, Mills SD, Pigazzi A, Nguyen NT, et al. Preoperative dehydration increases risk of postoperative acute renal failure in colon and rectal surgery. Journal of Gastrointestinal Surgery. 2014;**18**(12):2178-2185. Available from: https://pubmed.ncbi.nlm.nih.gov/25238816/

[5] Kaye A, anesthesia JRM, 2010 undefined. Intravascular fluid and electrolyte physiology. cir.nii.ac.jp Available from: https://cir.nii.ac.jp/crid/1361418519271313280

[6] Gurgel ST, Do Nascimento P. Maintaining tissue perfusion in high-risk surgical patients: A systematic review of randomized clinical trials. Anesthesia and Analgesia. 2011;**112**(6):1384-1391. Available from: https://pubmed.ncbi.nlm.nih.gov/21156979/

[7] Hamilton MA, Cecconi M, Rhodes A. A systematic review and meta-analysis on the use of preemptive hemodynamic intervention to improve postoperative outcomes in moderate and high-risk surgical patients. Anesthesia and Analgesia. 2011;**112**(6):1392-1402. Available from: https://pubmed.ncbi.nlm.nih.gov/20966436/

[8] Kendrick J, Kaye A, Tong Y, Belani K, Urman R, Hoffman C, et al. Goal-directed fluid therapy in the perioperative setting. Journal of Anaesthesiology Clinical Pharmacology. 2019;**35**(Suppl. 1):29-34. Available from: https://pubmed.ncbi.nlm.nih.gov/31142956/

[9] Bruegger D, Jacob M, Rehm M, Loetsch M, Welsch U, Conzen P, et al. Atrial natriuretic peptide induces shedding of endothelial glycocalyx in coronary vascular bed of Guinea pig hearts. American Journal of Physiology-Heart and Circulatory Physiology. 2005;**289**(5):1993-1999. Available from: https://journals.physiology.org/doi/abs/10.1152/ajpheart.00218.2005

[10] Jacob M, Chappell D, Hofmann-Kiefer K, Conzen P, Rehm M. A rational approach to perioperative fluid management. Anesthesiology. 2008;**109**(4):723-740. Available from: https://pubmed.ncbi.nlm.nih.gov/18813052/

[11] Kobe J, Mishra N, Arya VK, Al-Moustadi W, Nates W, Kumar B. Cardiac output monitoring: Technology and choice. Annals of Cardiac Anaesthesia. 2019;**22**(1):6-17. Available from: https://pubmed.ncbi.nlm.nih.gov/30648673/

[12] Rollins KE, Lobo DN. Intraoperative goal-directed fluid therapy in elective major abdominal surgery: A meta-analysis of randomized controlled trials. Annals of Surgery. 2016;**263**(3):465-476. Available from: https://pubmed.ncbi.nlm.nih.gov/26445470/

[13] Che L, Zhang XH, Li X, Zhang YL, Xu L, Huang YG. Outcome impact of individualized fluid management during spine surgery: A before-after prospective comparison study. BMC Anesthesiology. 2020;**20**(1):1-7. Available from: https://pubmed.ncbi.nlm.nih.gov/32698766/

[14] Chong MA, Wang Y, Berbenetz NM, McConachie I. Does goal-directed haemodynamic and fluid therapy improve peri-operative outcomes?: A systematic review and meta-analysis. European Journal of Anaesthesiology. 2018;**35**(7):469-483. Available from: https://pubmed.ncbi.nlm.nih.gov/29369117/

[15] Giglio M, Manca F, Dalfino L, Anestesiologica NBM. Perioperative hemodynamic goal-directed therapy and mortality: A systematic review and meta-analysis with meta-regression. Minerva Anestesiologica. 2016;**82**(11):1199-1213. Available from: https://europepmc.org/article/med/27075210

[16] Göçmen D, Köksal C, Abitağaoğlu S, Yildirim Ar A. Comparison of the effects of intraoperative goal directed and conventional fluid management on the inferior vena cava collapsibility index and postoperative complications in geriatric patients operated from proximal femoral nail surgery. Turkish Journal of Geriatrics. 2023;**26**(1):37. Available from: https://openurl.ebsco.com/contentitem/doi:10.29400%2Ftjgeri.2023.329?sid=ebsco:plink:crawler&id=ebsco:doi:10.29400%2Ftjgeri.2023.329

[17] Funk DJ, Moretti EW, Gan TJ. Minimally invasive cardiac output monitoring in the perioperative setting. Anesthesia and Analgesia. 2009;**108**(3):887-897. Available from: https://pubmed.ncbi.nlm.nih.gov/19224798/

[18] Guerin L, Monnet X, Teboul JL. Monitoring volume and fluid responsiveness: From static to dynamic indicators. Best Practice & Research. Clinical Anaesthesiology. 2013;**27**(2):177-185. Available from: https://pubmed.ncbi.nlm.nih.gov/24012230/

[19] Hasanin A. Fluid responsiveness in acute circulatory failure. Journal of Intensive Care. 2015;**3**(1):1-8. Available from: https://pubmed.ncbi.nlm.nih.gov/26594361/

[20] Michard F, Giglio MT, Brienza N. Perioperative goal-directed therapy with uncalibrated pulse contour methods: Impact on fluid management and postoperative outcome. British Journal of Anaesthesia. 2017;**119**(1):22-30. Available from: https://pubmed.ncbi.nlm.nih.gov/28605442/

[21] Marik PE, Monnet X, Teboul JL. Hemodynamic parameters to guide fluid therapy. Annals of Intensive Care. 2011;**1**(1):1-9. Available from: https://pubmed.ncbi.nlm.nih.gov/21906322/

[22] Le Manach Y, Hofer CK, Lehot JJ, Vallet B, Goarin JP, Tavernier B, et al. Can changes in arterial pressure be used to detect changes in cardiac output during volume expansion in the perioperative period? Anesthesiology. 2012;**117**(6):1165-1174. Available from: https://pubmed.ncbi.nlm.nih.gov/23135262/

[23] Lopes MR, Oliveira MA, Pereira VOS, Lemos IPB, Auler JOC, Michard F. Goal-directed fluid management based on pulse pressure variation monitoring

during high-risk surgery: A pilot randomized controlled trial. Critical Care. 2007;**11**(5):1-9. Available from: https://ccforum.biomedcentral.com/articles/10.1186/cc6117

[24] Berkenstadt H, Margalit N, Hadani M, Friedman Z, Segal E, Villa Y, et al. Stroke volume variation as a predictor of fluid responsiveness in patients undergoing brain surgery. Anesthesia and Analgesia. 2001;**92**(4):984-989. Available from: https://pubmed.ncbi.nlm.nih.gov/11273937/

[25] Guinot PG, De Broca B, Abou Arab O, Diouf M, Badoux L, Bernard E, et al. Ability of stroke volume variation measured by oesophageal doppler monitoring to predict fluid responsiveness during surgery. British Journal of Anaesthesia. 2013;**110**(1):28-33. Available from: https://pubmed.ncbi.nlm.nih.gov/22918700/

[26] Khwannimit B, Bhurayanontachai R. Prediction of fluid responsiveness in septic shock patients: Comparing stroke volume variation by FloTrac/Vigileo and automated pulse pressure variation. European Journal of Anaesthesiology. 2012;**29**(2):64-69. Available from: https://pubmed.ncbi.nlm.nih.gov/21946822/

[27] Reuter DA, Kirchner A, Felbinger TW, Weis FC, Kilger E, Lamm P, et al. Usefulness of left ventricular stroke volume variation to assess fluid responsiveness in patients with reduced cardiac function. Critical Care Medicine. 2003;**31**(5):1399-1404. Available from: https://pubmed.ncbi.nlm.nih.gov/12771609/

[28] Biais M, Nouette-Gaulain K, Cottenceau V, Revel P, Sztark F. Uncalibrated pulse contour-derived stroke volume variation predicts fluid responsiveness in mechanically ventilated patients undergoing liver transplantation. British Journal of Anaesthesia. 2008;**101**(6):761-768. Available from: https://pubmed.ncbi.nlm.nih.gov/18852114/

[29] Ramsingh DS, Sanghvi C, Gamboa J, Cannesson M, Applegate RL. Outcome impact of goal directed fluid therapy during high risk abdominal surgery in low to moderate risk patients: A randomized controlled trial. Journal of Clinical Monitoring and Computing. 2013;**27**(3):249-257. Available from: https://pubmed.ncbi.nlm.nih.gov/23264068/

[30] De Backer D, Heenen S, Piagnerelli M, Koch M, Vincent JL. Pulse pressure variations to predict fluid responsiveness: Influence of tidal volume. Intensive Care Medicine. 2005;**31**(4):517-523. Available from: https://pubmed.ncbi.nlm.nih.gov/15754196/

[31] Muller L, Bobbia X, Toumi M, Louart G, Molinari N, Ragonnet B, et al. Respiratory variations of inferior vena cava diameter to predict fluid responsiveness in spontaneously breathing patients with acute circulatory failure: Need for a cautious use. Critical Care. 2012;**16**(5):1-7. Available from: https://pubmed.ncbi.nlm.nih.gov/23043910/

[32] Monnet X, Bleibtreu A, Ferré A, Dres M, Gharbi R, Richard C, et al. Passive leg-raising and end-expiratory occlusion tests perform better than pulse pressure variation in patients with low respiratory system compliance. Critical Care Medicine. 2012;**40**(1):152-157. Available from: https://pubmed.ncbi.nlm.nih.gov/21926581/

[33] De Backer D, Taccone FS, Holsten R, Ibrahimi F, Vincent JL. Influence of respiratory rate on stroke volume variation in mechanically ventilated patients. Anesthesiology. 2009;**110**(5):1092-1097. Available

from: https://pubmed.ncbi.nlm.nih.gov/19352152/

[34] Monnet X, Osman D, Ridel C, Lamia B, Richard C, Teboul JL. Predicting volume responsiveness by using the end-expiratory occlusion in mechanically ventilated intensive care unit patients. Critical Care Medicine. 2009;**37**(3):951-956. Available from: https://pubmed.ncbi.nlm.nih.gov/19237902/

[35] Teboul J, Monnet X. Pulse pressure variation and ARDS. Minerva Anestesiologica. 2013;**79**(4):398-407. Available from: https://europepmc.org/article/med/23370121

[36] Vincent J, Weil MH. Fluid challenge revisited. Critical Care Medicine. 2013;**34**(5):1333-1337. Available from: https://journals.lww.com/ccmjournal/fulltext/2006/05000/fluid_challenge_revisited.5.aspx

[37] Muller L et al. An increase in aortic blood flow after an infusion of 100 ml colloid over 1 minute can predict fluid responsiveness: The mini-fluid challenge study. The Journal of the American Society of Anesthesiologists. 2011;**115**(3):541-547. DOI: 10.1097/ALN.0b013e318229a500. Available from: https://pubs.asahq.org/anesthesiology/article-abstract/115/3/541/11167

[38] Monnet X, Teboul JL. Passive leg raising. Intensive Care Medicine. 2008;**34**(4):659-663. Available from: https://pubmed.ncbi.nlm.nih.gov/18214429/

[39] Boulain T, Achard JM, Teboul JL, Richard C, Perrotin D, Ginies G. Changes in BP induced by passive leg raising predict response to fluid loading in critically ill patients. Chest. 2002;**121**(4):1245-1252. Available from: https://pubmed.ncbi.nlm.nih.gov/11948060/

[40] Dellinger RP, Levy M, Rhodes A, Annane D, Gerlach H, Opal SM, et al. Surviving sepsis campaign: International guidelines for management of severe sepsis and septic shock, 2012. Intensive Care Medicine. 2013;**39**(2):165-228. Available from: https://pubmed.ncbi.nlm.nih.gov/23361625/

[41] Cavallaro F, Sandroni C, Marano C, La Torre G, Mannocci A, De Waure C, et al. Diagnostic accuracy of passive leg raising for prediction of fluid responsiveness in adults: Systematic review and meta-analysis of clinical studies. Intensive Care Medicine. 2010;**36**(9):1475-1483. Available from: https://pubmed.ncbi.nlm.nih.gov/20502865/

[42] Monnet X, Rienzo M, Osman D, Anguel N, Richard C, Pinsky MR, et al. Passive leg raising predicts fluid responsiveness in the critically ill. Critical Care Medicine. 2006;**34**(5):1402-1407. Available from: https://pubmed.ncbi.nlm.nih.gov/16540963/

[43] De Backer D, Pinsky MR. Can one predict fluid responsiveness in spontaneously breathing patients? Intensive Care Medicine. 2007;**33**(7):1111-1113. Available from: https://pubmed.ncbi.nlm.nih.gov/17508200/

[44] Mahjoub Y, Touzeau J, Airapetian N, Lorne E, Hijazi M, Zogheib E, et al. The passive leg-raising maneuver cannot accurately predict fluid responsiveness in patients with intra-abdominal hypertension. Critical Care Medicine. 2010;**38**(9):1824-1829. Available from: https://pubmed.ncbi.nlm.nih.gov/20639753/

[45] Zhang Q, Wang X, Su L, Zhang H, Chai W, Chao Y, et al. Relationship between inferior vena cava diameter ratio and central venous pressure. Journal of

Clinical Ultrasound. 2018;**46**(7):450-454. Available from: https://pubmed.ncbi.nlm.nih.gov/29527693/

[46] Airapetian N, Maizel J, Alyamani O, Mahjoub Y, Lorne E, Levrard M, et al. Does inferior vena cava respiratory variability predict fluid responsiveness in spontaneously breathing patients? Critical Care. 2015;**19**(1)

[47] Orso D, Paoli I, Piani T, Cilenti FL, Cristiani L, Guglielmo N. Accuracy of ultrasonographic measurements of inferior vena cava to determine fluid responsiveness: A systematic review and meta-analysis. Journal of Intensive Care Medicine. 2020;**35**(4):354-363. Available from: https://pubmed.ncbi.nlm.nih.gov/29343170/

[48] Long E, Oakley E, Duke T, Babl FE. Does respiratory variation in inferior vena cava diameter predict fluid responsiveness: A systematic review and meta-analysis. Shock. 2017;**47**(5):550-559. Available from: https://pubmed.ncbi.nlm.nih.gov/28410544/

[49] Preau S, Bortolotti P, Colling D, Dewavrin F, Colas V, Voisin B, et al. Diagnostic accuracy of the inferior vena cava collapsibility to predict fluid responsiveness in spontaneously breathing patients with sepsis and acute circulatory failure. Critical Care Medicine. 2017;**45**(3):e290-e297. Available from: https://pubmed.ncbi.nlm.nih.gov/27749318/

[50] Prada G, Vieillard-Baron A, Martin AK, Hernandez A, Mookadam F, Ramakrishna H, et al. Echocardiographic applications of M-mode ultrasonography in anesthesiology and critical care. Journal of Cardiothoracic and Vascular Anesthesia. 2019;**33**(6):1559-1583

[51] Ceruti S, Anselmi L, Minotti B, Franceschini D, Aguirre J, Borgeat A, et al. Prevention of arterial hypotension after spinal anaesthesia using vena cava ultrasound to guide fluid management. British Journal of Anaesthesia. 2018;**120**(1):101-108. Available from: https://pubmed.ncbi.nlm.nih.gov/29397116/

[52] Ciozda W, Kedan I, Kehl DW, Zimmer R, Khandwalla R, Kimchi A. The efficacy of sonographic measurement of inferior vena cava diameter as an estimate of central venous pressure. Cardiovascular Ultrasound. 2015;**14**(1):1-8. Available from: https://pubmed.ncbi.nlm.nih.gov/27542597/

[53] Brennan JM, Blair JE, Goonewardena S, Ronan A, Shah D, Vasaiwala S, et al. Reappraisal of the use of inferior vena cava for estimating right atrial pressure. Journal of the American Society of Echocardiography. 2007;**20**(7):857-861. Available from: https://pubmed.ncbi.nlm.nih.gov/17617312/

[54] Lang RM, Badano LP, Victor MA, Afilalo J, Armstrong A, Ernande L, et al. Recommendations for cardiac chamber quantification by echocardiography in adults: An update from the American Society of Echocardiography and the European Association of Cardiovascular Imaging. Journal of the American Society of Echocardiography. 2015;**28**(1):1-39.e14. Available from: https://pubmed.ncbi.nlm.nih.gov/25559473/

[55] Marik PE, Cavallazzi R, Vasu T, Hirani A. Dynamic changes in arterial waveform derived variables and fluid responsiveness in mechanically ventilated patients: A systematic review of the literature. Critical Care Medicine. 2009;**37**(9):2642-2647. Available from: https://pubmed.ncbi.nlm.nih.gov/19602972/

[56] Weinberg L, Harris L, Bellomo R, Ierino FL, Story D, Eastwood G, et al.

Effects of intraoperative and early postoperative normal saline or Plasma-Lyte 148® on hyperkalaemia in deceased donor renal transplantation: A double-blind randomized trial. British Journal of Anaesthesia. 2017;**119**(4):606-615. Available from: https://pubmed.ncbi.nlm.nih.gov/29121282/

[57] Yunos NRAM, Bellomo R, Hegarty FC, Story D, Ho L, Bailey M. Association between a chloride-liberal vs chloride-restrictive intravenous fluid administration strategy and kidney injury in critically ill adults. JAMA. 2012;**308**(15):1566-1572. Available from: https://pubmed.ncbi.nlm.nih.gov/23073953/

[58] O'Malley CMN, Frumento RJ, Hardy MA, Benvenisty AI, Brentjens TE, Mercer JS, et al. A randomized, double-blind comparison of lactated Ringer's solution and 0.9% NaCl during renal transplantation. Anesthesia and Analgesia. 2005;**100**(5):1518-1524. Available from: https://pubmed.ncbi.nlm.nih.gov/15845718/

[59] Neto AS, Loeches IM, Klanderman RB, Silva RF, de Abreu MG, Pelosi P, et al. Balanced versus isotonic saline resuscitation-a systematic review and meta-analysis of randomized controlled trials in operation rooms and intensive care units. Annals of Translational Medicine. 2017;**5**(16). Available from: https://pubmed.ncbi.nlm.nih.gov/28861420/

[60] Bampoe S, Odor PM, Dushianthan A, Bennett-Guerrero E, Cro S, Gan TJ, et al. Perioperative administration of buffered versus non-buffered crystalloid intravenous fluid to improve outcomes following adult surgical procedures. Cochrane Database of Systematic Reviews. 2017;**9**(9). Available from: https://pubmed.ncbi.nlm.nih.gov/28933805/

[61] Krajewski ML, Raghunathan K, Paluszkiewicz SM, Schermer CR, Shaw AD. Meta-analysis of high- versus low-chloride content in perioperative and critical care fluid resuscitation. The British Journal of Surgery. 2015;**102**(1):24-36. Available from: https://pubmed.ncbi.nlm.nih.gov/25357011/

[62] McFarlane C, Lee A. A comparison of Plasmalyte 148 and 0.9% saline for intra-operative fluid replacement. Anaesthesia. 1994;**49**(9):779-781. Available from: https://pubmed.ncbi.nlm.nih.gov/7978133/

[63] Annane D, Siami S, Jaber S, Martin C, Elatrous S, Declère AD, et al. Effects of fluid resuscitation with colloids vs crystalloids on mortality in critically ill patients presenting with hypovolemic shock: The CRISTAL randomized trial. JAMA. 2013;**310**(17):1809-1817. Available from: https://pubmed.ncbi.nlm.nih.gov/24108515/

[64] Lewis SR, Pritchard MW, Evans DJW, Butler AR, Alderson P, Smith AF, et al. Colloids versus crystalloids for fluid resuscitation in critically ill people. Cochrane Database of Systematic Reviews. 2018;**8**(8). Available from: https://pubmed.ncbi.nlm.nih.gov/30073665/

[65] Navickis RJ, Haynes GR, Wilkes MM. Effect of hydroxyethyl starch on bleeding after cardiopulmonary bypass: A meta-analysis of randomized trials. The Journal of Thoracic and Cardiovascular Surgery. 2012;**144**(1):223-230. Available from: https://pubmed.ncbi.nlm.nih.gov/22578894/

[66] Kulemann B, Timme S, Seifert G, Holzner PA, Glatz T, Sick O, et al. Intraoperative crystalloid overload leads to substantial inflammatory infiltration of intestinal anastomoses-a

histomorphological analysis. Surgery. 2013;**154**(3):596-603. Available from: https://pubmed.ncbi.nlm.nih.gov/23876362/

[67] Marjanovic G, Villain C, Juettner E, Zur HA, Hoeppner J, Hopt UT, et al. Impact of different crystalloid volume regimes on intestinal anastomotic stability. Annals of Surgery. 2009;**249**(2):181-185. Available from: https://pubmed.ncbi.nlm.nih.gov/19212167/

[68] Holte K, Kehlet H. Fluid therapy and surgical outcomes in elective surgery: A need for reassessment in fast-track surgery. Journal of the American College of Surgeons. 2006;**202**(6):971-989. Available from: https://pubmed.ncbi.nlm.nih.gov/16735213/

[69] Holte K, Sharrock NE, Kehlet H. Pathophysiology and clinical implications of perioperative fluid excess. British Journal of Anaesthesia. 2002;**89**(4):622-632. Available from: https://pubmed.ncbi.nlm.nih.gov/12393365/

[70] Siparsky N, com/contents RSO de https://www. uptodate, 2017 undefined. Overview of postoperative fluid therapy in adults [Internet]. 2017. Available from: https://www.uptodate.com/contents/overview-of-postoperative-fluid-therapy-in-adults; https://medilib.ir/uptodate/show/15073 [Accessed: May 27, 2024]

[71] Tazreean R, Nelson G, Twomey R. Early mobilization in enhanced recovery after surgery pathways: Current evidence and recent advancements. Journal of Comparative Effectiveness Research. 2022;**11**(2):121-129. Available from: https://pubmed.ncbi.nlm.nih.gov/35045757/

Chapter 3

Perspective Chapter: Anaesthetic Management for Robotic Surgery

Amr Ashour, Ahmed Aboelezz, Mohamed Hussein, Mustafa Rehan and Belal Khalil

Abstract

Robotic surgery has been widely adopted by many centres as it provides optimum surgical conditions for management of various cases with improved outcomes over the past decade. Being a relatively new technique, anaesthesia for robotic surgery has become a part of daily work that anaesthetists should know about. This chapter aims to provide a comprehensive review about latest advances in robotic surgeries, indications, and contraindication, the perioperative management plan, and recent techniques to provide pain relief for intra- and postoperative care focusing on the latest PROSPECT guidelines. It will highlight the possible complications that should always be kept in mind during and after surgery period.

Keywords: robotic surgery, preoperative assessments, intraoperative managements, postoperative complications, pain management, PROSPECT guidelines

1. Introduction

1.1 History of robotic-assisted devices in medicine

The field of medicine is undergoing a revolution with the emergence of robots. Various factors such as miniaturisation, artificial intelligence, and computer power are helping in the design and development of these robotic systems [1].

About 34 years ago, medical robots started to emerge when a CT navigation system and an industrial robot were used to carry out a biopsy procedure on the brain. Eventually, medical robots were able to perform various surgical procedures, such as total hip arthroplasty and urological procedures. Unfortunately, these fully autonomous robots were not popular with surgeons [1].

The technology drew the attention of the US Department of Defence, which invested in it to allow performing surgeries over troop casualties without jeopardising the medical team using satellites. The project faced various technical issues, mainly due to the delay in response time. However, the project facilitated the development of the Da Vinci System which was introduced to the medical system in 1999 [1].

1.2 Surgeries and robotic-assisted devices

In the past few decades, surgical techniques have witnessed major changes from open techniques towards minimally invasive ones, saving patients a large, traumatic, and painful incision. Not only positively affecting the patients but also saving costs from prolonged hospital stay and recovery time [1].

The evolution of minimally invasive techniques using small cameras did not pass without a cost. The two-dimensional (2D) flattened visual operative field limited the surgical techniques and flexibility until 1985, when the robot PUMA 560 performed a CT-guided brain biopsy that opened a new world of minimally invasive techniques, allowing better 3D visual field surgeries [1].

1.3 The Da Vinci System

The Da Vinci System comprises three parts: a console, a robotic manipulator, and a visualising tower. The console consists of an eyepiece giving 3D image, two actuators controlling the robot's arms and foot pedals allowing change between control of camera and robotic arms and changing the diathermy power. The visualising tower carries images from the camera to display to the theatre team. The robotic manipulator consists of three arms; one holds the camera, and the other two carry different surgical instruments. The camera is slightly different from the endoscopic camera as it contains two cameras that fuse the images together to give the surgeon a 3D image with real depth. The system has advanced technology to filter hand tremors and allows precise movement. Moreover, instrument arms have a higher degree of free mobility than conventional laparoscopic arms to approximate the human hand's range of movement (**Figure 1**) [2].

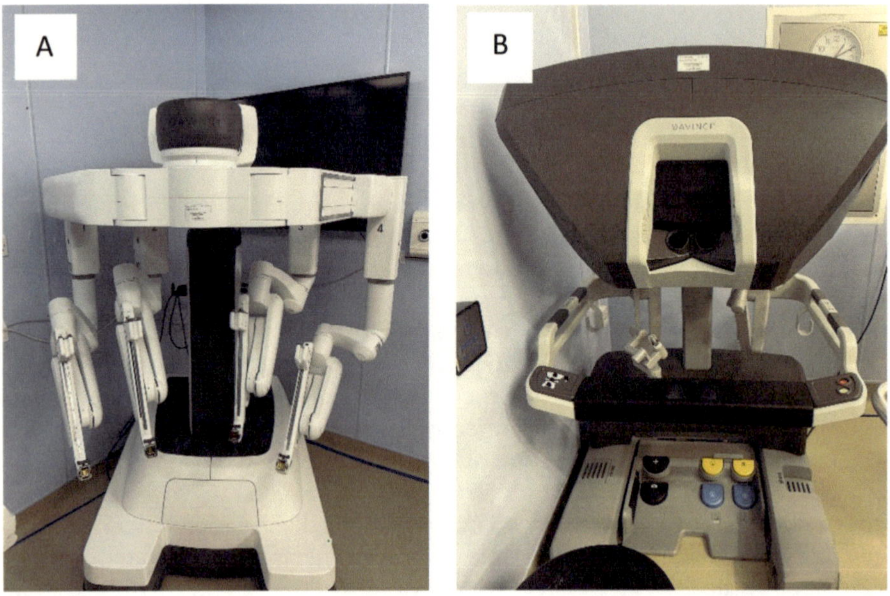

Figure 1.
The Da Vinci robot (a) console (b) robotic manipulator and visualising tower—Southend University Hospitals NHS Trust Theatre.

In spite of the advanced technology of the Da Vinci System, it has its drawbacks. The system requires a surgeon to insert the robotic arms through a laparoscopic-sized hole. So, remote surgery is still possible but needs a surgeon in the field. The Da Vinci System is a relatively new technology costing around 1.5 million Pound with yearly service of around 125 thousand and 2000 Pound per case, which is considered a high cost for most of the UK trusts [3]. However, the high cost could be equilibrated with the lower cost of hospital stay after the surgery and lower incidence of complications that have been reported especially with the use of robotic surgery in prostatectomy. Moreover, the learning curve of robotic surgeries is relatively long when compared with laparoscopic surgeries, for example, which is time-consuming and may result in prolonged surgeries, also reflected in the cost of robotic surgery. Robotic surgery has an ergonomic issue and requires a spacious operating theatre with the theatre team, not only surgeons and anaesthetists, who are familiar with the procedure and machine. From an anaesthetic point of view, any patient movement could lead to a disastrous result once the robotic arms are locked inside the patient's body, requiring complete muscle relaxation [4].

The Da Vinci System is reliable, with a failure rate leading to open surgery approaching 0.5%. The lower risks of postoperative complications have led to a global shift towards robotic surgeries [4, 5]. A study published in the *Journal of American Medical Association* regarding robotic surgeries for bladder cancer and reconstruction has found a reduced chance for re-admission by 52%, quicker recovery by 20%, and reduced prevalence of blood clots (deep venous thrombosis (DVT) and pulmonary emboli) by 77%. The system has been introduced to various surgical specialities including general, cardiothoracic, gynaecological, paediatric, neurological, and recently urological surgeries [6].

1.4 Pneumoperitoneum

Pneumoperitoneum is required to facilitate robotic surgery. As the name suggests, the gas used in pneumoperitoneum is carbon dioxide (CO_2). CO_2 has multiple advantages to be used in pneumoperitoneum rather than air or any other gas. CO_2 is an inert gas that does not readily undergo chemical reactions with other substances and does not support combustion that will allow the safe use of diathermy. It also has a significant solubility, decreasing the risk of gas embolism if injected into a blood vessel mistakenly [7, 8].

There are multiple considerations that should be kept in mind due to pneumoperitoneum. The abdomen and the pelvis are relatively closed spaces, and when the gas is injected, it will lead to increased intra-abdominal pressure (IAP). At the start, the movement of the diaphragm and the anterior abdominal wall will accommodate for the increased IAP. With increased pressure, the compensatory mechanism will fail, resulting in a rapid increase in the IAP. The sequela of the increased IAP is compression of the inferior vena cava, major arteries, and visceral blood vessels. That will lead to decreased venous return to the heart, dropping the cardiac output (COP) and pooling of blood in the abdomen, facilitating the development of deep venous thrombosis. The raised IAP will also be reflected in increased pressure on other closed spaces such as the brain leading to increased intracranial tension (ICT) [9].

The change in IAP is biphasic: A mild increase in the IAP (<10 mmHg) will lead to an increase in venous return, causing elevation in COP and blood pressure. Further, an increase in IAP (10–20 mmHg) will reduce COP and increase systemic vascular resistance, which will be reflected variably in blood pressure. When IAP is raised above 20 mmHg, the drop in COP becomes significant, leading to a drop in blood pressure [10].

Pneumoperitoneum also affects respiratory function by splitting the diaphragm, leading to basal atelectasis affecting the ventilation/perfusion matching. The CO_2 is absorbed into the circulation by the large peritoneal surface, even after deflation, leading to a rise in arterial CO_2, reducing the partial pressure of O_2 in alveoli [11].

In addition to previous changes, pneumoperitoneum increases the pressure on the small blood vessels supplying the viscera. A relatively small rise in IAP from 10 to 15 mmHg significantly affects the blood supply to stomach, liver, and small and large intestines, increasing the risk of ischaemic injury. The retroperitoneal structures are relatively preserved; however, there is a reduction in renal blood flow, resulting in an alteration of renal function [12].

The effects of pneumoperitoneum are exaggerated by the change in position. Trendelenburg position will add to the negative effect exerted on lungs; however, it will improve the venous return. On the other hand, the reverse Trendelenburg position will reserve the venous return but will deteriorate the respiratory function [13, 14].

2. Preoperative considerations of robotic surgery

2.1 Common indications of robotic surgery in the practice

Robotic techniques have become standard practice in urology, particularly for procedures like prostatectomy, uncomplicated adrenalectomy, and nephrectomy, including live donor nephrectomy. In gynaecologic surgery, robotics play a crucial role in procedures such as tubal surgery (sterilisation, treatment of ectopic pregnancy, etc.), cystectomies, hysterectomies, various ablations (endometriosis), and more. Robotic surgery is also applied during pregnancy and in paediatric cases [15].

The realm of robotic general surgery encompasses a wide range of procedures, including cholecystectomy, hernia repair, anti-reflux procedures, splenectomy, appendectomy, bowel surgery (including bariatric procedures), and various upper and lower abdominal interventions. Recent advancements extend the application of robotics to thoracoscopic, cardiovascular, and neurosurgical intracranial surgeries, utilising modified laparoscopic instruments without the need for gas insufflation [16].

Additionally, emerging trends include lumbar discectomies and other forms of spinal surgery performed laparoscopically through an anterior approach. Remarkably, even autopsies have been explored using laparoscopic techniques. The ongoing expansion of robotic applications in diverse medical fields continues to broaden the scope of minimally invasive procedures [16].

2.2 Contraindication of robotic surgeries

Most of the contra-indications of robotic surgeries could be reverted by surgical team experience. However, contra-indications of robotic surgery should be excluded during preoperative assessment as robotic surgeries are better avoided in these conditions [17].

Contra-indications of robotic surgery could be divided based on systems:

- CNS: increased intracranial pressure, space-occupying lesion, retinal detachment, acute glaucoma, shunts (at risk of gas emboli and shunt obstruction).

- Cardiorespiratory: severe cardiovascular or pulmonary disease, hypovolemic shock, bullae, severe right, or biventricular failure, right to left cardiac shunt.

- Renal: impending renal shutdown.

- Abdominal: peritonitis, large intra-abdominal mass, abdominal wall tumour, history of extensive surgery or adhesions, diaphragmatic hernia, morbid obesity.

- Haematological: coagulopathy, sickle cell disease (risk of precipitation of sickle cell crisis with acidosis).

To summarise, contra-indications are related to the ability of the patient to tolerate extremes of position, pneumoperitoneum, and hypercarbia. It is worth mentioning that pregnancy is no longer considered a contraindication for robotic surgery, provided that the anaesthetist keeps in mind the effect of robotic surgery on maternal and fetal changes. Arterial gas monitoring with pre and postoperative fetal and uterine monitoring is essential [17].

2.3 Preoperative assessment

Vigilant assessment of the cardiopulmonary system is mandatory in preoperative assessment due to the reasons mentioned before. The effect of age on pulmonary function should always be kept in mind as with increased age, the functional residual capacity (FRC) decreases. Smoking and chronic obstructive pulmonary disease (COPD) cause a higher secretion with decreased ciliary clearance function, leading to further issues in ventilation added to the effect of pneumoperitoneum together, which may deteriorate the respiratory function. Respiratory infection might have a detrimental effect on intraoperative respiratory function and should be excluded until management with appropriate antibiotics. High BMI and deviation of the spine (Kyphoscoliosis) will add to the issues related to respiratory function. Assessment of exercise tolerance and the presence of shortness of breath will help in the formulation of plan of management. Thorough airway assessment should be considered especially if the patient is undergoing transoral robotic surgery (TORS). Difficult airway and obstructive sleep apnoea (OSA) are always considered in these types of surgeries [17].

Basic preoperative tests should be ordered in preoperative assessment including complete blood count, clotting functions, chemistry, electrolytes, renal function, ECG blood typing, and screening. Other laboratory tests may be required depending on the history taken. Baseline pulmonary function tests, chest X-ray, arterial blood gas, and saturation on room air might be helpful in patients with pulmonary diseases. Echocardiography, cardiac stress test, and cardiology clearance might be required for patients with cardiological symptoms [7].

Patients should be informed of possible complications of surgery as usual. He should be aware of the possibility of emergency laparotomy with possible blood transfusion and intensive care unit admission. Preoperative bowel preparation and antibiotics could be required before surgery in some surgical intervention.

3. Intraoperative considerations of robotic surgery

3.1 Anaesthetic technique

General anaesthesia with cuffed endotracheal tube insertion with controlled positive pressure ventilation is the recommended technique for robotic surgery. This can be explained by the long duration of the procedure, the extreme positions, the need to insert nasogastric or orogastric tubes and the need for muscle relaxation. The need for muscle relaxation is extremely important for robotic surgery as the increased intra-abdominal pressure with splinting of the diaphragm makes spontaneous breathing difficult. Moreover, any patient movement after docking the robot could lead to outrageous consequences. Also, muscle relaxation is useful to allow augmentation of ventilation to decrease levels of CO_2 associated with abdominal insufflation [5].

The successful use of laryngeal mask (LMA) in some short laparoscopic procedures has been reported. However, the limited capability of applying positive pressure ventilation and the insecure guarding against aspiration in robotic surgery contraindicates its usage in robotic surgery [18].

Regional anaesthesia alone could be used successfully in laparoscopic surgery, but it is impossible to use alone in robotic surgery due to the positioning, the high sensory block level required, and the hyperventilation required to maintain a normal level of CO_2. Besides, the patient's tolerance to a long procedure such as robotic surgery is questionable. Regional anaesthesia can be combined with general anaesthesia for pain relief. However, it should be kept in mind that the sympathetic response to abdominal insufflation, which maintains the blood pressure and cardiac output, will be abolished by regional anaesthesia [19, 20].

Any combination of anaesthetic agents that provides amnesia, analgesia, and paralysis could be used. The use of antiemetics is recommended, as peritoneal stimulation and distension will increase the risk of postoperative nausea and vomiting (PONV). A combined use of antiemetics of different mechanisms of action is advised. The choice between inhalational anaesthetics and total intravenous anaesthesia (TIVA) is operator-dependent as long as guarding against awareness is kept in mind using the required level of monitoring (end-tidal inhalational level and/or Bispectral Index). The use of nitrous oxide is controversial due to its diffusion capability, bowel distension causing more difficulties in surgery and postoperative nausea and vomiting [7].

3.2 Monitoring and access

The level of monitoring for robotic surgery can differ from one patient to another depending on the patient's comorbidities, degree of complexity, and length of surgical procedure and expected blood loss. Generally speaking, many anaesthetists prefer invasive arterial lines for monitoring blood pressure and frequent gas analysis besides the standard monitoring (ECG, oximeter, capnogram, inspired O_2 fraction, end-tidal inhalational anaesthetic, minute ventilation, peak airway pressure, urine output, and oesophageal temperature monitor). However, it should always be kept in mind that access to the patient during surgery is extremely limited. So, lines should always be secured with extra caution. Line kinking, displacement, and obstruction are common issues during robotic surgery due to the fact that access is limited, especially after docking of the robot. EEG monitoring is preferable in some conditions when there is a risk of postoperative cognitive dysfunction to avoid unnecessarily deep levels of anaesthesia.

Usually, standard IV access with wide-bore cannulae would be enough to maintain anaesthesia and intraoperative fluid therapy. However, central venous pressure (CVP), pulmonary artery pressure, pulmonary artery occlusion pressure (PAOP), and cardiac output should be used in some patients depending on their comorbidities [21–23].

3.3 Positioning

Positioning in robotic surgery is one of the major factors that affects patient condition. In robotic surgery, extreme forms of Trendelenburg and reverse Trendelenburg are not uncommon. Also, it should be kept in mind that changing the position after docking the robot is difficult. The position effect on patient health can be summarised as follows [7]:

- Respiratory: movement of endotracheal tube and bronchial intubation, airway oedema, atelectasis, aspiration.

- Cardiovascular: reduced venous return and hypotension.

- Central nervous system: cerebral and conjunctival oedema, C5-7 disruption.

- Peripheral nervous system: compression on various nerves depending on position, neuropraxia, neuropathy.

- Gastrointestinal: increased risk of reflux and mouth ulcers (from acid reflux).

- Musculoskeletal: pressure sores, compartment syndrome.

Measures to avoid complications related to position can be summarised as follows [7]:

- Delicate positioning with gel padding, straps with support and avoidance of stretching of limbs and compression stocking.

- Good securing of the cuffed endotracheal tube with a recheck of its position after patient positioning and avoidance of tight ties. Check the cuff pressure after inflation and consider a leak test before extubation.

- Usage of positive end-expiratory pressure (PEEP).

- Insertion and drainage of nasogastric tube.

- Preload the patient with fluids, make judicious fluid intake, and consider the usage of vasopressors before positioning.

- Periodic checking of the patient face.

3.4 Ventilation

Lung protective ventilation has been suggested for ventilation in robotic surgery. However, there is no available data for the best PEEP level to be used. High PEEP levels would provide better lung aeration. On the other hand, it will negatively affect blood pressure and increase the risk of barotrauma and alveolar overdistension. Lower PEEP levels will avoid these problems. Various studies tried to find the best PEEP level. From these studies, we can conclude that zero-end expiratory pressure should be avoided, and moderate PEEP levels (4–8 cmH_2O) have been associated with better outcomes than high PEEP levels (>10 cmH_2O). However, an individualised PEEP level is optimal [24].

No specific data is available to define the best mode of ventilation independently from other ventilatory parameters. It is suggested to set the tidal volume to 6–8 ml/kg of predicted body weight with a PEEP level of 4–8 cmH_2O. However, it is suggested to use pressure-controlled ventilation with a monitor of tidal volume to avoid barotrauma and better gas exchange. Inspiratory:expiratory ratio of 2:1 or 1:1 has been found to improve CO_2 clearance through decreasing dead space fraction. Although prolonged inspiratory time has been found beneficial for acute lung injury patients by improving oxygenation, no such effect has been noticed in robotic surgery [25].

Recruitment manoeuvres are frequently used to decrease atelectasis, improve alveolar ventilation, and decrease intrapulmonary shunting. However, it might decrease venous return and lead to barotrauma and alveolar overdistension. It is better to be used in case of hypoxemia or deterioration of respiratory mechanics during or after pneumoperitoneum [26].

3.5 Intravenous fluids

IV fluid management in robotic surgery is an art balance between maintaining perfusion and preventing volume overload. Recent surgical practice results in euvolemic patients preoperatively by carbohydrate loading, reduced bowel preparation, and reduced fluid fasting hours.

A relatively new concept in fluid management is introduced depending on the delivery of O_2 (DO_2) divided by body surface area to produce indexed oxygen delivery (DO_2I) measured by ml/min/m^2. Multiple literature can be found supporting the idea that maintaining high DO_2I has an effect on decreasing morbidity and mortality in open surgeries. However, the effect of robotic surgeries needs further investigation [27].

The advised approach to fluid management is [5]:

- Fluid replacement for pre-existing fluid deficit if present.
- Targeting zero fluid balance with maintenance around 1–4 ml/kg/h and replacement of measured losses.
- Intraoperative hypotension should be managed with vasopressors rather than fluids unless it is due to hypovolemia.

- Monitoring of urinary output is required, especially in prolonged complex robotic surgery. Permissive oliguria with urine output of 0.3 ml/kg/h is widely adopted without affection of renal function.

- CVP is inaccurate in the management of fluid balance due to the extremes of position and pneumoperitoneum. Other markers such as serum lactate, acid-base balance, and central venous oxygen saturation provide better monitoring of fluid status.

The increased risk of cerebral oedema, especially in extreme Trendelenburg positions, should always be kept in mind while managing the fluid status of the patient.

3.6 Analgesia

Multimodal analgesia with opioid-sparing drugs is the new trend in the analgesic management of surgical operations. Large doses of opioids are associated with a higher incidence of postoperative nausea and vomiting, suppression of cough reflex, delay in return of gastrointestinal (GIT) function, and higher risk for opioid misuse [28].

Epidural analgesia for such operations was considered the gold standard for a long time. However, due to causes related to delayed return of GIT function, reduced mobility, increased fluid requirement, and increased hospital stay, the use of epidural analgesia is declining when compared with single-shot spinal anaesthesia and morphine PCA [29].

A popular method of injection of 250–1000 mcg of intrathecal diamorphine with regular postoperative paracetamol and non-steroidal anti-inflammatory drugs (NSAIDs), unless contraindicated, is used with reserving of opioid use to breakthrough pain [5]. The usage of other regional techniques such as transversus abdominis block (TAP), especially before the operation starts was successful. Some practitioners use remifentanil infusion to manage some physiological responses during surgery. However, there are still some concerns about tolerance and hyperalgesia [30].

The second line of analgesics using IV ketamine and lidocaine is currently under focus, especially for IV lidocaine and its role in decreasing postoperative nausea and vomiting and opioid use. However, the exact timing, dosing, and duration of IV lidocaine are still inconclusive [31, 32].

3.7 Muscle relaxants

Muscle relaxation in robotic surgery is mandatory to prevent patient coughing and movement. Multiple comparisons between a deep level of relaxation (post-tetanic count of one to two twitches) and a moderate level of relaxation (train of four of one to two twitches) have been made. Theoretically, a deep level of relaxation will provide better surgical conditions with lower intra-abdominal pressure (8–15 mmHg). However, the difference between the two levels is still not obvious [5].

3.8 Antiemetics

Usage of multi-modal antiemetics in robotic surgery is advised due to the higher risk of postoperative nausea and vomiting associated with robotic surgery [5].

4. Intraoperative complications of robotic surgery

4.1 Cardiovascular complications

Cardiovascular complications during robotic surgery could be generally considered uncommon. Bradycardia that might develop asystole due to abdominal insufflation is the commonest [33]. Other complications include arrhythmia, atrial fibrillation, bundle branch block, cardiogenic pulmonary oedema, and, less commonly, myocardial ischaemia and infarction [34–36].

4.2 Vascular complications

The most devastating vascular complication related to robotic surgery is lower limb compartment syndrome, with an incidence of 0.02%. The management is usually fluid resuscitation and analgesics, and sometimes might need bilateral fasciotomy. Lower limb compartment syndrome could be explained by increased intra-abdominal pressure, lithotomy position, and Trendelenburg position that led to decreased blood flow to lower limbs [11].

Venous gas embolism is one of the common vascular complications of robotic surgery with an incidence of 7–10%. However, mostly, it has no cardiovascular effect or other sequelae. That could be explained by the Trendelenburg position and increased right atrial pressure that guards against the haemodynamic effect [11].

Other vascular complications include deep venous thrombosis, vascular injury, especially during port insertion, and rhabdomyolysis, which is commonly associated with compartment syndrome [11].

4.3 Cardiac arrest and robot failure

Please refer to chapter (Perioperative considerations for patients undergoing robotic radical prostatectomy).

5. Postoperative complications of robotic surgery

The advantages of robotic surgery cannot be ignored. On the other hand, with the emergence of robotic surgery, multiple changes and complications were noted affecting all systems of the human body. Complications were noted from case reports and case series after the introduction of robotic surgery. It could be categorised according to the system affected:

5.1 Neurological complications

Most complications related to robotic surgery are neurological, and a good percentage of them are related mainly to positioning. It could be further subdivided into central and peripheral nervous system complications [11].

Cerebral oedema is the main central nervous system complication. It could lead to a postoperative altered mental state that sometimes needs reintubation. Cerebral oedema is related to the Trendelenburg position and increased intra-abdominal pressure. Both factors would lead to increased central venous pressure and capillary leak. Preventive measures could be limiting time for steep Trendelenburg position, limiting operative time, fluid restriction, and limiting intra-abdominal pressure to 8 mmHg as possible. Cerebral oedema could be managed using dexamethasone and diuretics [37–40].

Peripheral nerve damage is relatively uncommon but devastating, commonly related to steep Trendelenburg position and long operative time. The mechanism of injury could be explained by stretch, ischaemia, and compression. The overall incidence of peripheral nerve injury in robotic surgery is 0.25% [41].

Upper extremities nerve injury is mainly brachial plexus injury with an incidence of 20% of all peripheral nerve injuries. The most common nerve injury is ulnar nerve followed by the brachial plexus and median nerve. The injury could be related to pressure over acromioclavicular joints. Fortunately, most upper extremity injuries have no long-term sequelae and resolve spontaneously within a few weeks [42–48].

Lower extremity nerve injury could be related to steep Trendelenburg with lithotomy position. This position could lead to compression of the peroneal nerve between head of fibula and leg support and compression of the saphenous nerve against the medial tibial condyle. Furthermore, other lower limb nerves could be affected by this position such as obturator nerve, common peroneal nerve, sciatic nerve, and lateral femoral cutaneous nerve. Lower limb nerve injury incidence ranges between 0.3% and 5.1% [49–51].

5.2 Ophthalmic complications

The most common ophthalmic complication is corneal abrasion which could be related to incomplete coverage of the eye and conjunctival oedema. Other complications include ischaemic optic neuropathy and various degrees of visual field affection and blindness [11].

5.3 Pulmonary complications

Pulmonary complications related to robotic surgery could be summarised in basal atelectasis as a result of abdominal insufflation and Trendelenburg position, hypoxemia due to migration of endotracheal tube to the right main bronchus, aspiration with microaspiration being more common, airway oedema, and pneumothorax [11].

5.4 Renal complications

Renal complications ranged from mild elevation of renal function up to acute kidney injury (AKI). The incidence of acute kidney injury in robotic surgery versus open surgery is still controversial. Acute kidney injury could be noted in the form of oliguria <0.5 ml/kg/h for >6 hours or elevation in serum creatinine. Acute kidney injury could be explained by elevated abdominal pressure, which leads to increased renal vascular resistance being more common in the elderly. Others suggest that the reason could be rhabdomyolysis and compartment syndrome. Oliguria without clinical manifestations has been reported and could be attributed to renal compression [52–57].

5.5 Gastrointestinal complications

Few complications were noted in the gastrointestinal system and could be considered nonspecific to robotic surgery. One case report of acute hepatic injury could be explained by increased intra-abdominal pressure leading to portal ischaemia. Small bowel and colon damage during port insertion has also been reported [58, 59].

5.6 Musculoskeletal complications

Musculoskeletal complications could be divided into trauma, subcutaneous emphysema, and oedema. Trauma has been noticed in multiple areas of the body including face, digits thigh, flanks, oral ulceration, and subconjunctival. Cervical and lumbar strain was also noted without long-term sequelae, though. Moreover, pressure sores are reported commonly in the gluteal area with various degrees, and vacuum mattresses should be considered, especially in prolonged procedures [11].

Subcutaneous emphysema has been reported relatively frequently. Some reports referred to mediastinal emphysema but without long-term effects. Risk factors for developing subcutaneous emphysema could be prolonged operative time, increased $etCO_2 > 5.3$ kPa and more than five surgical ports [11].

Postoperative conjunctival oedema is very common, and some consider it a common effect of steep Trendelenburg. Significant oedema in multiple body parts was also noted in a fair number of cases, while the incidence of head and neck oedema reached 12%, which could lead to airway oedema and delay of extubation and, in some cases, reintubation [11].

6. PROSPECT guidelines for postoperative pain management in radical prostatectomy

Procedure-specific postoperative pain management (PROSPECT) is a guideline developed by a group of anaesthetists and surgeons in order to manage postoperative pain in radical prostatectomy (open, laparoscopic, or robotic) and is updated based on systematic review and meta-analysis. M. Lemoine and colleagues published PROSPECT guidelines in Anaesthesia and Critical Care Medicine, 2021 that concluded [60]:

1. Comprehensive pain relief should involve the administration of paracetamol and either selective or non-selective nonsteroidal anti-inflammatory drugs before or during surgery, with ongoing postoperative continuation.

2. During open surgery, it is advisable to employ continuous intravenous lidocaine. However, its usage contradicts the concurrent use of local anaesthetics through infiltration.

3. In the absence of intravenous lidocaine usage, local wound infiltration should be routinely employed for open surgery before considering other regional analgesia blocks.

4. For laparoscopic/robotic radical prostatectomy, it is recommended to prioritise the Transversus Abdominis Plane block as a plan of analgesia.

5. In the postoperative period, opioids are recommended for use as rescue analgesics.

7. Conclusion

The emergence of robotic surgery might someday change the shape of medicine that we know. The advantages of robotic surgery outweigh its drawbacks. Being a relatively new technique, robotic surgery is still under continuous development. Anaesthetic management of robotic surgery could be challenging given the physiological changes related to position, duration of surgery, and abdominal insufflation. Various anaesthetic techniques have been developed to manage such cases. However, complications of robotic surgery could not be ignored, and the ultimate aim for anaesthesia is to provide a safe patient journey through the surgery.

Acknowledgements

The authors would like to thank Southend University Hospital NHS Trust for providing an image of the Di Vinci robotic system.

Conflict of interest

The authors declare no conflict of interest.

Author details

Amr Ashour[1*], Ahmed Aboelezz[2], Mohamed Hussein[3], Mustafa Rehan[4] and Belal Khalil[5]

1 Milton Keynes University Hospital, UK

2 Conquest Hospital, UK

3 Ashford and St Peter Hospitals, UK

4 Royal Lancaster Infirmary, UK

5 Southend University Hospital, UK

*Address all correspondence to: amr.ashour@mkuh.nhs.uk

References

[1] Sandham J. Robotic assisted surgery. Electrical and Biomedical Engineering EBME. EBME and Clinical Engineering articles [Internet]. Available from: https://www.ebme.co.uk/articles/clinical-engineering/robotic-assisted-surgery

[2] Irvine M, Patil V. Anaesthesia for robot-assisted laparoscopic surgery. Continuing Education in Anaesthesia, Critical Care & Pain. 2009;**9**(4):125-129

[3] Ashrafian H et al. The evolution of robotic surgery: Surgical and anaesthetic aspects. British Journal of Anaesthesia. 2017;**119**(Supplement 1):172-184

[4] Zorn KC, Gofrit ON, Orvieto MA, Mikhail AA, Galocy RM, Shalhav AL, et al. Da Vinci robot error and failure rates: Single institution experience on a single three-arm robot unit of more than 700 consecutive robot-assisted laparoscopic radical prostatectomies. Journal of Endourology. 2007;**21**(11):1341-1344

[5] Carey BM et al. Anaesthesia for minimally invasive abdominal and pelvic surgery. British Journal of Anaesthesia Education. 2019;**19**(8):254-260

[6] Catto JW, Khetrapal P, Ricciardi F, Ambler G, Williams NR, Al-Hammouri T, et al. Effect of robot-assisted radical cystectomy with intracorporeal urinary diversion vs open radical cystectomy on 90-day morbidity and mortality among patients with bladder cancer: A randomized clinical trial. Journal of the American Medical Association. 2022;**327**(21):2092-2103

[7] Weingram J. Robotic-assisted laparoscopic surgery. In: Yao F et al., editors. Yao & Artusio's Anesthesiology Problem-oriented Patient Management. 9th ed. Philadelphia: Wolter Kluwer; 2021. pp. 1433-1492

[8] Menes T, Spivak H. Laparoscopy "Searching for the proper insufflation gas" Presented at the meeting of the Society of American Gastrointestinal Endoscopic Surgeons (SAGES), San Antonio, Texas, USA, March 1999. Surgical Endoscopy. 2000;**14**:1050-1056

[9] Chiumello D et al. Ventilation strategy during urological and gynaecological robotic-assisted surgery: A narrative review. British Journal of Anaesthesia. 2023;**131**(4):764-774

[10] Neudecker J, Sauerland S, Neugebauer E, Bergamaschi R, Bonjer HJ, Cuschieri A, et al. The European Association for Endoscopic Surgery clinical practice guideline on the pneumoperitoneum for laparoscopic surgery. Surgical Endoscopy. 2002;**16**:1121-1143

[11] Maerz DA et al. Complications of robotic-assisted laparoscopic surgery distant from the surgical site. British Journal of Anaesthesia. 2017;**118**(4):492-503

[12] O'Malley C, Cunningham AJ. Physiologic changes during laparoscopy. Anesthesiology Clinics of North America. 2001;**9**(1):1-9

[13] Grabowski JE, Talamini MA. Physiological effects of pneumoperitoneum. Journal of Gastrointestinal Surgery. 2009;**13**:1009-1016

[14] Hatipoglu S, Akbulut S, Hatipoglu F, Abdullayev R. Effect of laparoscopic abdominal surgery on splanchnic

circulation: Historical developments. World Journal of Gastroenterology: WJG. 2014;**20**(48):18165

[15] Muñoz CJ, Nguyen HT, Houck CS. Robotic surgery and anesthesia for pediatric urologic procedures. Current Opinion in Anaesthesiology. 2016;**29**(3):337-344

[16] Efron DT, Bender JS. Laparoscopic surgery in older adults. Journal of the American Geriatrics Society. 2001;**49**(5):658-663

[17] Vinod M, Anuj M, Anup P, Daniel G. Anesthesia and the renal and genitourinary system. In: Gropper MA, Eriksson LI, Fleisher LA, Wiener-Kronish JP, Cohen NH, Leslie K, editors. Miller's Anesthesia, 2-Volume Set. 9th ed. Philadelphia, PA: Elsevier - Health Sciences Division; 2019. pp. 1929-1959

[18] Bapat PP, Verghese C. Laryngeal mask airway and the incidence of regurgitation during gynecological laparoscopies. Anesthesia & Analgesia. 1997;**85**(1):139-143

[19] Collins LM, Vaghadia H. Regional anesthesia for laparoscopy. Anesthesiology Clinics of North America. 2001;**19**(1):43-55

[20] Vaghadia H, Solylo MA, Henderson CL, et al. Selective spinal anesthesia for outpatient laparoscopy. II: Epinephrine and spinal cord function. Canadian Journal of Anaesthesia. 2001;**48**:261-266

[21] Jacobs VR, Morrison JE Jr, Mettler L, et al. Measurement of CO_2 hypothermia during laparoscopy and pelviscopy: How cold it gets and how to prevent it? The Journal of the American Association of Gynecologic Laparoscopists. 1999;**6**:289-295

[22] Ogunnaike BO, Jones SB, Jones DB, et al. Anesthetic considerations for bariatric surgery. Anesthesia and Analgesia. 2002;**95**(6):1793-1805

[23] Tournadre JP, Chassard D, Berrada KR, et al. Effect of pneumoperitoneum and Trendelenburg position on gastro-oesophageal reflux and lower oesophageal sphincter pressure. British Journal of Anaesthesia. 1996;**76**:130-132

[24] Kim JY, Shin CS, Kim HS, et al. Positive end-expiratory pressure in pressure-controlled ventilation improves ventilatory and oxygenation parameters during laparoscopic cholecystectomy. Surgical Endoscopy. 2010;**24**(5):1099-1103

[25] Kim MS, Kim NY, Lee KY, et al. The impact of two different inspiratory to expiratory ratios (1:1 and 1:2) on respiratory mechanics and oxygenation during volume-controlled ventilation in robot-assisted laparoscopic radical prostatectomy: A randomized controlled trial. Canadian Journal of Anaesthesia. 2015;**62**(9):979-987

[26] Kim WH, Hahm TS, Kim JA, et al. Prolonged inspiratory time produces better gas exchange in patients undergoing laparoscopic surgery: A randomised trial. Acta Anaesthesiologica Scandinavica. 2013;**57**:613-622

[27] Ackland GL, Iqbal S, Paredes LG, Toner A, Lyness C, Jenkins N, et al. Individualised oxygen delivery targeted haemodynamic therapy in high-risk surgical patients: A multicentre, randomised, double-blind, controlled, mechanistic trial. The Lancet Respiratory Medicine. 2015;**3**(1):33-41

[28] Levy BF, Scott MJ, Fawcett W, Fry C, Rockall TA. Randomized clinical trial of epidural, spinal or patient-controlled

analgesia for patients undergoing laparoscopic colorectal surgery. The British Journal of Surgery. 2011;**98**:1068-1078

[29] Levy BF, Scott MJ, Fawcett WJ, Rockall TA. 23-hour-stay laparoscopic colectomy. Diseases of the Colon and Rectum. 2009;**52**:1239-1243

[30] De Oliveira GS, Castro-Alves LJ, Nader A, Kendall MC, McCarthy RJ. Transversus abdominis plane block to ameliorate postoperative pain outcomes after laparoscopic surgery: A meta-analysis of randomized controlled trials. Anesthesia and Analgesia. 2014;**118**:454-463

[31] Ventham NT, Kennedy ED, Brady RR, et al. Efficacy of intravenous lidocaine for postoperative analgesia following laparoscopic surgery: A meta-analysis. World Journal of Surgery. 2015;**39**:2220e34 21

[32] Weibel S, Jelting Y, Pace NL, et al. Continuous intravenous perioperative lidocaine infusion for postoperative pain and recovery in adults. Cochrane Database of Systematic Reviews. 2018;**6**:CD009642

[33] Gainsburg DM. Anesthetic concerns for robotic-assisted laparoscopic radical prostatectomy. Minerva Anestesiologica. 2012;**78**:596-604

[34] Sharma A, Berkeley A. Intraoperative drug-eluting stent thrombosis in a patient undergoing robotic prostatectomy. Journal of Clinical Anesthesia. 2009;**21**:517-520

[35] Lee LC. Cardiopulmonary collapse in the wake of robotic surgery. AANA Journal. 2014;**82**:231-234

[36] Thompson J. Myocardial infarction and subsequent death in a patient undergoing robotic prostatectomy. AANA Journal. 2009;**77**:365-371

[37] Pandey R, Garg R, Darlong V, et al. Unpredicted neurological complications after robotic laparoscopic radical cystectomy and ileal conduit formation in steep Trendelenburg position: Two case reports. Acta Anaesthesiologica Belgica. 2010;**61**:163-166

[38] Barr C, Madhuri TK, Prabhu P, Butler-Manuel S, Tailor A. Cerebral oedema following robotic surgery: A rare complication. Archives of Gynecology and Obstetrics. 2014;**290**:1041-1044

[39] Kakar PN, Das J, Roy PM, Pant V. Robotic invasion of operation theatre and associated anaesthetic issues: A review. Indian Journal of Anaesthesia. 2011;**55**:18-25

[40] Kaye AD, Vadivelu N, Ahuja N, et al. Anesthetic considerations in robotic-assisted gynecologic surgery. The Ochsner Journal. 2013;**13**:517-524

[41] Berger J, Alshaeri T, Lukula D, Dangerfield P. Anesthetic considerations for robot-assisted gynecologic and urology surgery. Journal of Anesthesia & Clinical Research. 2013;**4**:345

[42] Gupta K, Mehta Y, Sarin Jolly A, Khanna S. Anaesthesia for robotic gynaecological surgery. Anaesthesia and Intensive Care. 2012;**40**:614-621

[43] Lee JR. Anesthetic considerations for robotic surgery. Korean Journal of Anesthesiology. 2014;**66**:3-11

[44] Devarajan J, Byrd JB, Gong MC, et al. Upper and middle trunk

brachial plexopathy after robotic prostatectomy. Anesthesia & Analgesia. 2012;**115**:867-870

[45] Ulm MA, Fleming ND, Rallapali V, et al. Position-related injury is uncommon in robotic gynecologic surgery. Gynecologic Oncology. 2014;**135**:534-538

[46] Hsu RL, Kaye AD, Urman RD. Anesthetic challenges in robotic-assisted urologic surgery. Revista de Urología. 2013;**15**:178-184

[47] McLarney JT, Rose GL. Anesthetic implications of robotic gynecologic surgery. International Journal of Gynecological Endoscopy. 2011;**2**:75-78

[48] Kalmar AF, De Wolf AM, Hendrickx JF. Anesthetic considerations for robotic surgery in the steep Trendelenburg position. Advances in Anesthesia. 2011;**1**:75-96

[49] Gezginci E, Ozkaptan O, Yalcin S, et al. Postoperative pain and neuromuscular complications associated with patient positioning after robotic assisted laparoscopic radical prostatectomy: A retrospective non-placebo and nonrandomized study. International Urology and Nephrology. 2015;**47**:1635-1641

[50] Koc G, Tazeh NN, Joudi FN, et al. Lower extremity neuropathies after robot-assisted laparoscopic prostatectomy on a split-leg table. Journal of Endourology. 2012;**26**:1026-1029

[51] Awad H, Walker CM, Shaikh M, et al. Anesthetic considerations for robotic prostatectomy: A review of the literature. Journal of Clinical Anesthesia. 2012;**24**:494-504

[52] Romagnoli S, Zagli G, Tuccinardi G, et al. Postoperative acute kidney injury in high-risk patients undergoing major abdominal surgery. Journal of Critical Care. 2016;**35**:120-569

[53] Lim SY, Lee JY, Yang JH, et al. Predictive factors of acute kidney injury in patients undergoing rectal surgery. Kidney Research and Clinical Practice. 2016;**35**:160-164

[54] Joo EY, Moon YJ, Yoon SH, et al. Comparison of acute kidney injury after robot-assisted laparoscopic radical prostatectomy versus retropubic radical prostatectomy: A propensity score matching analysis. Medicine (Baltimore). 2016;**95**:2650

[55] Herling SF, Havemann MC, Palle C, Moller AM, Thomsen T. Robotic-assisted laparoscopic hysterectomy seems safe in women with early-stage endometrial cancer. Danish Medical Journal. 2015;**62**:A5109-A5172

[56] Galyon SW, Richards KA, Pettus JA, Bodin SG. Three-limb compartment syndrome and rhabdomyolysis after robotic cystoprostatectomy. Journal of Clinical Anesthesia. 2011;**23**:75-78

[57] Chiu AW, Chang LS, Birkett DH, Babayan RK. The impact of pneumoperitoneum, pneumoretroperitoneum, and gasless laparoscopy on the systemic and renal hemodynamics. Journal of the American College of Surgeons. 1995;**181**:397-406

[58] Karadag MA, Cecen K, Demir A, et al. Gastrointestinal complications of laparoscopic/robot-assisted urologic surgery and a review of the literature. Journal of Clinical Medical Research. 2015;**7**:203-210

[59] Jakimowicz J, Stultiens G, Smulders F. Laparoscopic insufflation of

the abdomen reduces portal venous flow. Surgical Endoscopy. 1998;**12**:129-132

[60] Lemoine M et al. PROSPECT guidelines update for evidence based pain management after prostatectomy for cancer. Anaesthesia Critical Care and Pain Medicine. 2021;**40**(4):100922

Chapter 4

Perspective Chapter: Perioperative Considerations for Patients Undergoing Robotic Radical Prostatectomy

Amandeep Virk, Victor Yu, Wenjie Zhong, Samuel Davies and Scott Leslie

Abstract

Robotic radical prostatectomy has become the dominant surgical approach for men with clinically localized prostate cancer, surpassing open and laparoscopic techniques. The robotic platform offers magnified, stereoscopic vision, and endo-wristed instruments to improve surgical dissection and suturing which enhances patient outcomes. The minimally invasive approach offers similar oncological and functional results to the open procedure, but has the advantage of reduced hospital length of stay, shorter catheter time and fewer complications. These important gains in patient care can be maximized with a complete understanding of the relevant perioperative considerations. The outcomes and patient experience for men undergoing robotic radical prostatectomy can be maximized with a careful and personalized approach that is integrated into their care before, during and after surgery.

Keywords: perioperative, robotic surgery, prostatectomy, prostate cancer, Trendelenburg, pneumoperitoneum, lithotomy, anesthetics

1. Introduction

Prostate cancer is the second most prevalent male malignancy worldwide, with approximately 1.4 million new cases diagnosed annually [1]. Its prevalence increases with age and contributes a significant health burden globally. Robotic assisted prostatectomy has become the preferred option for the management of localized prostate cancer. Robotic surgery offers the advantages of minimally invasive surgery whilst providing better access and dexterity within the confined limits of the pelvis. Yaxley et al. found robotic assisted radical prostatectomy (RARP) to have shorter operative times, less blood loss and lower rates of intraoperative complications when compared to open prostatectomy in their landmark paper [2, 3]. The paper also found patients who underwent RARP had less post operative pain at early time points and shorter stays in hospital and that there long-term functional and oncological outcomes were similar [2, 3]. With further technological advancements and techniques combined with improved surgical experience, the robotic approach to prostatectomy will gain further advantages.

In this chapter, we delve into the pertinent peri-operative considerations for patients who are undergoing RARP. Focus will be directed towards pre-operative optimization, patient selection, intra-operative preparation, access and standards of post-operative management.

2. Pre-operative considerations

2.1 Patient selection

Radical prostatectomy is a treatment option for patient with localized prostate cancer, along with external beam radiation therapy, brachytherapy, and in some cases active surveillance. Preoperative counseling should include both the patient, and where relevant, their support person to address the practical and emotional issues surrounding radical prostatectomy. Presurgical psychosocial interventions may be useful in improving quality of life following surgery. In addition, patients should be counseled regarding modification of high-risk health behaviors such as smoking and weight loss.

The selection of patients includes an assessment of the patient's physical health and function, a discussion about goals of care and potential adverse outcomes.

Patients are assessed for life expectancy as curative treatments including RARP, are generally offered to patients who have an estimated life expectancy of greater than 10–15 years.

Specifically, assessment includes; co-morbidities, nutrition, cognition and function. These parameters can be associated with overall survival, rates of return to baseline function and risks of post-operative adverse events such as delirium and extended hospitalization [4, 5]. Other considerations include extensive previous surgery, which may present a technical challenge due to adhesions.

For patients for whom there is concern regarding physical and cognitive function, a formal physician assessment may be beneficial. A range of screening scores are used in assessing overall health, including the Geriatric 8 (G8) screening tool and the Clinical Frailty Scale (CFS). In particular, the G8 score is useful in discriminating between fit and frail patients, with frail patients at higher risk of mortality and treatment related morbidity [6]. Current guidelines from the European Association of Urology (EAU) recommends the use of these scales prior to treatment of prostate cancer, as well as the use of comprehensive geriatric assessment for patients who are at high risk (e.g. patients with G8 score ≤ 14) [7].

Although the standard recommendations for curative treatment for prostate cancer is an estimated life expectancy of greater than 10 years, there is increasing evidence that older patients are under-treated and have potential benefit from robotic prostatectomy. Patients over 75, in several retrospective trials have shown similar functional and oncological outcomes compared to their younger counterparts, suggesting a select proportion of healthy, elderly prostate cancer patients can be offered treatment [8, 9]. In any case, decision to proceed with RARP should be shared. The patients' values and preferences need to be considered in addition to objective function assessment.

2.2 Neo-adjuvant therapy

The use of neo-adjuvant androgen deprivation therapy (ADT) has been the focus of several randomized controlled trials. Although histopathological improvements have been demonstrated (including downstaging, reduced positive margins and lower incidence of positive lymph nodes), clinical oncological parameters of PSA-relapse free survival and cancer specific survival remained static [10]. These findings, supported by a systematic review and meta-analysis, affirm that the use of neo-adjuvant ADT is not routinely recommended prior to radical prostatectomy [11]. However, with the introduction of novel antiandrogens (daralutomide, enzalutamide), there are clinical trials currently underway, assessing the oncological benefits for men receiving these drugs in the neoadjuvant setting [12]. Furthermore, the impact that these drugs have on perioperative outcomes, such as complications and length of hospital stay, is another important consideration that these trials will shed light on.

2.3 Anesthetic considerations

Patients undergoing RARP should be pre-operatively screened with a thorough medical history and physical examination. Focus should be drawn to any cardiac and respiratory history, including the regular use of anticoagulation or antiplatelets, diabetes, obesity, reflux, and renal abnormalities (especially in the context of prostatic obstruction).

General cardiac risk should be assessed at the time of pre-operative screening to determine the need for further investigations and management to reduce the risk of cardiac complications. History of ischaemic heart disease, congestive heart failure, cerebral vascular disease, renal dysfunction, and pre-operative insulin treatment are all indicators of high cardiac risk [13].

An important consideration for anesthesia in RARP is the combination of high intra-abdominal pressures due to the pneumoperitoneum and the steep Trendelenburg positioning [14]. Patients at particularly high risk in this context include cardio-respiratory conditions (**Table 1**), morbid obesity, raised intracranial pressure (ICP) and glaucoma [15]. The specifics of intra-operative management of these will be discussed later in this chapter.

At our institution, the pre-operative anesthetic assessment includes electrocardiogram, full blood count, electrolytes, and chest X-ray. Men with high-risk co-morbidities are referred to relevant specialists to ensure they are maximally optimized prior to

Absolute contraindications
Metastatic prostate cancer
Life expectancy <10 years
Active peritoneal inflammatory process
Relative contraindications
Morbid obesity
Extensive peritoneal, perineal, or pelvic surgery
Glaucoma

Table 1.
Absolute and relative contraindications for robotic radical prostatectomy.

High risk co-morbidities in robotic prostatectomy
• *Severe or decompensated heart failure (both left and right sided)*
• *Severe valvular disease (particularly aortic stenosis)*
• *Significant arrhythmias*
• *Ischaemic heart disease (including recent myocardial infarction, angina)*
• Severe respiratory disease (particularly COPD, poorly controlled asthma, pulmonary hypertension)

Table 2.
High risk co-morbidities in robotic prostatectomy. Patients with any of the above cardiac conditions (italicized) are recommended by AHA/ACC guidelines to have either delay or cancelation of non-emergent procedures [13].

the procedure. If perioperative risks are considered too great, then alternative forms of treatment for their cancer may be necessary (**Table 2**).

2.4 Obesity and weight loss

As with other abdominal or pelvic procedures, obesity remains a technical challenge for the surgeon during RARP. Obesity in RARP can result in reduced overall working space, difficulties with trocar placement, reduced intra-peritoneal vision and anesthetics risks. Obesity is associated with higher complication rates as compared to normal weight controls [16].

Patients are encouraged and provided with strategies to reduce weight prior to surgery. In our institution, we often recommend low calorie diet plans for patients with a body max index over 30 kg/m^2. We utilize Optifast very low calorie diet program which is a commercially available meal replacement product plan with less than 800 calories per day. This can be associated weight loss of 1–2.5 kg per week [17]. Pharmacological therapy with Semaglutide, a glucagon-like peptide-1 (GLP-1), is a recently available option which has proven efficacious for weight loss in obese patients which can be considered when available [18].

Simultaneously, the operating team should be aware of the physical limitations and potential complications that accompany obese patients, and appropriate adjustments and preparations made. Although obesity can make RARP challenging, the access that the robotic camera and instruments allow into the deep pelvis, permits the surgical removal of the prostate where it would not have been possible with conventional open or laparoscopic techniques.

2.5 Patient education and preparation

Important patient outcomes following RARP is the return of continence and erectile function. Intra-operative techniques such as nerve-sparing, bladder slings [19] and specific re-anastomosis sutures [20] have allowed for improvements in functional recovery and will be discussed further separately. The use of pre-operative pelvic floor exercises can optimize the recovery of these functional deficits, particularly incontinence. One systematic review and meta-analysis has shown an improved rate of return of continence post-radical prostatectomy [21]. However, there is a lack of uniformity in the regimens used as well as the definitions of continence. Pelvic floor exercise regimes are commenced 1 month prior to surgery and patients are instructed to continue post-operatively. This is run by a specialist pelvic floor physiotherapist to educate on appropriate exercises. This is supplemented by biofeedback and pelvic floor ultrasound to help patients recruit the appropriate pelvic floor muscles.

During the pre-operative period, patients should be provided with education about the procedure itself. This gives the opportunity to discuss expectations and most importantly, a shared, informed consent can be obtained. Patient understanding has been demonstrated to improve long-term patient satisfaction following radical prostatectomy [22]. The use of adjuncts in this process including multi-media tools and 3D models further enhance patient understanding [23, 24].

2.6 Peri-procedural medications

The risk of withholding antiplatelet and anticoagulation must be weighed against their indications, particularly for patients with previous cardiac percutaneous interventions, metallic valve replacement and venous thromboembolism. An individualized medication plan is employed with discussion with other specialists if there is concern or the patient is high-risk. RARP can be safely performed on aspirin, but this is at the surgeon's discretion. A range of antiplatelet and anticoagulants and their cessation recommendations are listed in **Table 3** [25].

Diabetic patients need careful managed to optimize wound and anastomotic healing. It also reduces peri-procedural diabetic complications such as diabetic ketoacidosis, hyperglycaemic hyperosmolar state and severe hypoglycaemia in the fasting pre-operative patient. Regular diabetic medications are withheld the morning of surgery in the fasting patient. The increased use of sodium-glucose cotransporter 2 inhibitors (SGLT-2) has raised another issue of euglycemic diabetic ketoacidosis. These medications need to be withheld for at least 3 days.

Bowel preparation is not typically utilized prior to robotic prostatectomy, as the risk of rectal injury is low. The use of bowel preparation is considered in select cases such as salvage prostatectomy, when rectal injury is more likely [26].

2.7 Prostatectomy associated urinary tract infection

Prior to RARP, a urine microscopy and culture is sent to rule out urinary tract infection or asymptomatic bacteriuria. Our institution performs this at the pre anesthetic assessment, 1–2 weeks prior to procedure. This allows time for culture growth and sensitivities and appropriate antibiotic treatment.

Medication	Time to withhold prior to robotic prostatectomy
Enoxaparin	24 hours
NOACs (e.g. rivaroxaban, dabigatran, apixaban)	24–72 hours (depending on renal function)
NSAIDs, antiplatelets (e.g. aspirin)	5 days
Warfarin	5 days (with INR check 2 days prior to procedure)
Other antiplatelets (e.g. clopidogrel, ticagrelor)	7 days

Table 3.
Duration of withholding of common anticoagulants and antiplatelets prior to robotic prostatectomy. Adapted from Guidelines on Perioperative Management of Anticoagulation and Antiplatelet Agents, CEC [25].

3. Intra operative considerations

3.1 Patient positioning and room set up

Patient positioning and room ergonomics are critical when incorporating a robotic platform into the theater environment. The robotic platform consists of the surgeon's console, computer control tower, patient docking cart and viewing screens which all take up additional space and can limit patient access [27, 28].

Close communication between the surgeon and anesthetist ensures optimal patient positioning for operative efficiency. The most common positioning for RARP is lithotomy with Trendelenburg with the docking cart between the legs or at the patients' side [29].

In preparation for Trendelenburg, a non-slip foam mat may be used to prevent patient movement [27, 30]. This is important as once the robot arms are docked to the ports, movement can cause injury to the incision sites or result in instrument movement within the patient causing injury [27, 30, 31]. Other methods of securing the patient include straps or bolsters at the shoulders but we have found these additional methods to be unnecessary.

The patient's legs are placed in lithotomy stirrups. Care is taken to avoid extreme flexion of the hip or knees and ensure well-padded stirrups are used to reduce the risk of lower limb pressure areas or neuropraxia [32].

Peripheral access lines and pulse oximetry are well padded to prevent pressure areas and gel pads used to prevent pressure where the hand contacts the lithotomy stirrup. The arm should be secured in a relaxed and neutral position to reduce the risk of neuropraxia [30, 31]. We recommend the palm face the body with the thumbs up to reduce strain on the ulnar nerve. A method used in our institution is to use soft orthopedic padding to wrap the arms to prevent pressure areas from lines and the surroundings prior to securing the arm in position at the patients' side by using a pillowcase tucked underneath the patients' torso, around the arm and then back under the patient for loose but secure immobilization [33].

Once the patient is positioned and in the desired Trendelenburg position a final check is made prior to docking the robotic arms.

3.2 Monitoring and access

Careful arrangement of lines and monitoring is a critical concern for the anesthesiologist as there is less access once the patient is draped, and the robot docked. Access to the airway is also partially obstructed by the proximity of the robotic arms to the face. This is particularly relevant should emergent access be required to the face and chest area for cardiopulmonary resuscitation should the situation arise. For these reasons we also recommend the endotracheal tube is well secured and the face is protected to limit accidental contact with the robot [27].

3.3 Trendelenburg

RARP requires steep Trendelenburg positioning to optimize access and vision within the pelvis. The 20–30 degree Trendelenburg allows the bowel to drop cephalad out of the pelvic cavity, an affect which is more evident once any restricting abdominal adhesion are released [27, 30, 34]. In our institution we use a protractor to measure the Trendelenburg angle and ensure the minimal angle for the desired affect is used.

Trendelenburg position causes venous congestion leading to raised intraocular pressure (IOP) [35]. The raised IOP is time dependent and decreases when returned to the supine position [15, 35]. Normal IOP is 10–21 millimeters of mercury (mmHg) and pressures greater than 21 mmHg reduce ocular perfusion pressure and risks retinal detachment, post operative visual loss, glaucoma and ischemic optic neuropathy [15, 35]. The reduced venous return and increased episcleral venous pressure from pneumoperitoneum exacerbates this affect [36]. Propofol may reduce IOP compared to sevoflurane and neuromuscular blockade may also reduce IOP by aiding aqueous humor drainage by relaxing the extraocular musculature [34, 35].

The limited access to the face and proximity to the robotic arms in Trendelenburg can cause accidental contact to the patients face leading to corneal abrasion, the most common ocular complication [34]. A review of 1500 consecutive robotic assisted radical prostatectomies found a decrease in corneal abrasion from 3% to 1% with the use of eye patches instead of tapes [34, 37]. More recently, Trendelenburg positioning itself has also been shown to be a risk factor for corneal abrasion due to increased corneal thickness because of elevated intraocular and episcleral venous pressure and conjunctival oedema [34, 36, 38].

Trendelenburg combined with the effects of pneumoperitoneum increase intracranial pressure (ICP) [30, 34]. A proposed mechanism is the reduced drainage of the lumbar venous plexus and the vasodilatory effects of hypercarbia increasing cerebral blood volume and CSF volume [30]. The Monroe Kellie hypothesis explains an equilibrium between the CSF, blood volume and parenchymal tissue in the fixed space of the skull dictating a rise in ICP with a rapid rise in any of these constituents. Caution should be taken in patients with pre-existing intracranial hypertension or pathology [34, 39]. Despite the known increases in ICP, Weisinger et al. demonstrate no change in cerebral oxygenation during 45-degree Trendelenburg for procedures up to 5 hours in length and no change in post operative mental function as measured by a mini mental status examination [40].

We recommend careful control of CO_2 to maintain normocarbia, minimizing total time in Trendelenburg and minimize the angle used. Nishikawa et al. found performing RARP with a 25-degree angle compared to 30-degree angle of Trendelenburg reduced intraoperative IOP and did not increase operative time or estimated blood loss in their series of 30 cases [41]. Another proposed strategy by Raz et al. is a modified Z Trendelenburg position whereby the head and shoulders are elevated to the horizontal whilst in Trendelenburg (**Figure 1**) [42]. In their randomized control trial study, they found this modification reduced IOP and did not impact anesthesia, the procedure of the operative field [42].

3.4 Pneumoperitoneum

Abdominal CO_2 insufflation is used to create intra-abdominal working space. The pressures commonly used range from 12 to 15 mmHg [30, 34]. The European Association for Endoscopic Surgery recommend using the lowest possible pressure required for adequate vision of the surgical field [43].

The hemodynamic effects of pneumoperitoneum are dynamic when combined with steep Trendelenburg [30, 34, 44]. Mean arterial pressure (MAP) and systemic vascular resistance (SVR) increased with pneumoperitoneum [44]. This affect is

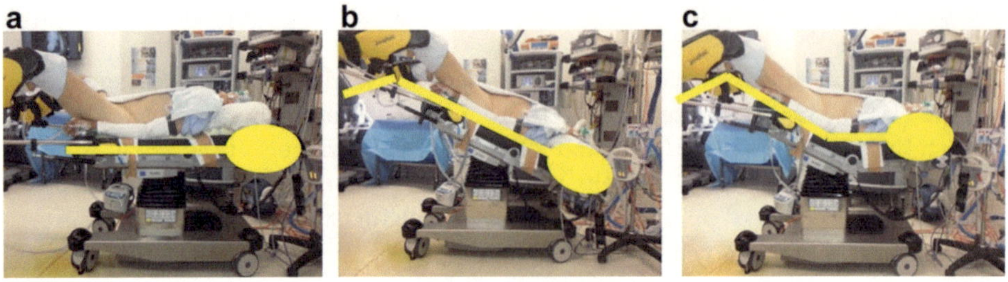

Figure 1.
Modified Z Trendelenburg position. Reproduced from Raz et al. [42]. a, horizontal supine position with lithotomy. b, 23-degree Trendelenburg position with lithotomy. c, modified Z Trendelenburg position.

produced from the increased afterload from intra-abdominal pressure causing local compression of the aorta as well as neurohumoral factors [30, 34]. When combined with Trendelenburg, SVR returns to basal levels but MAP remains elevated [44]. Trendelenburg also raises the CVP, the mean pulmonary artery pressure (MPAP) and the pulmonary capillary wedge pressure (PCWP) [44]. The net effect is a 25% increase in MAP, and a more than 2-fold increase in CVP, MPAP and CVP [44]. Heart rate, stroke volume and cardiac output were unchanged by these effects however the left ventricular stroke work index and right ventricular stroke work index increased by 35% and 65% respectively [44]. This indicated that cardiac function is maintained in the patient with cardiac reserve, but caution needs to be taken in patients with impaired baseline function [30, 34]. The observed hemodynamic changes all returned to baseline on exsufflation and returning to the horizontal position [44]. When treatment is required, the aim is often afterload reduction given this is a major component of the observed changes [45].

The cephalad displacement of the diaphragm by insufflation reduces lung functional reserve capacity (FRC) and decreases pulmonary compliance [30, 34]. The affect is compounded by the gravitational forces of the abdominal contents on the diaphragm and mediastinum from Trendelenburg positioning and associated raised pulmonary pressures [30, 34]. With a 11–12 mmHg insufflation pressure and 45-degree Trendelenburg, Lestar et al. measured a fall in total lung compliance from 60 to 28 mm/cm of water [44]. The net result is increased peak inspiratory pressures to maintain minute ventilation and the associated increased risk of barotrauma [30, 34].

The most practical remedy for hypercapnia from peritoneal CO_2 absorption is hyperventilation, however the increased peak inspiratory pressures need to be considered in increasing minute ventilation [27, 30, 39]. If normocapnia proves difficult to maintain, permissive hypercapnia may be considered, or alternatively temporary lowering of pneumoperitoneum pressures may be required to facilitate a period of hyperventilation [39].

Subcutaneous emphysema is a common complication of pneumoperitoneum which self resolves with exsufflation and is rarely of a magnitude to cause clinical concern as CO_2 is highly soluble when compared to air [30, 34, 45]. However, severe cases can cause hypercarbia complicating ventilation. If permissive hypercarbia is required to manage the resultant hypercarbia, the patient may benefit from remaining mechanically ventilated at the end of surgery until corrected to reduce an increased work of breathing [30, 39]. The other concern is for the spread of subcutaneous emphysema in pre fascial planes causing pneumothorax or pneumomediastinum [30, 45]. If there is subcutaneous emphysema extending to the thorax or neck, we recommend evaluation with mobile chest Xray. While CO_2 is rapidly absorbed into the bloodstream, large quantities could necessitate the need for surgical decompression with a chest tube [45].

Venous gas embolism is a life-threatening complication that should be suspected when there is unexplained cardiovascular collapse and correlating capnographic changes [30, 45]. High risk periods for gas entry into the circulation are during insufflation and ligation of the dorsal venous complex [30, 34]. It is not uncommon for the surgeon to use transiently higher insufflation pressures up to 20 mmHg during the dorsal veinous complex ligation to limit venous blood loss. While the rapid absorbability of CO_2 compared to air minimizes the risk of embolus, should clinically apparent gas embolus be suspected, insufflation should be immediately ceased [27, 45].

3.5 Ventilation

The requirements for paralysis, pneumoperitoneum and Trendelenburg to perform RARP necessitates general anesthesia with a cuffed endotracheal tube secured and mechanically ventilated [45]. Once the patient is positioned for docking, we recommend rechecking tube position. The cephalad pressure effect of pneumoperitoneum and Trendelenburg causes shortening of the trachea and can result in endobronchial intubation [30, 34, 46].

The establishment of pneumoperitoneum and Trendelenburg leads to increased airway pressures. A degree of ventilation difficulty should be expected in patients with chronic pulmonary disease or the morbidly obese [27, 45]. Managing peak airway pressure to prevent barotrauma while also regulating end tidal CO_2 to maintain normocapnia can be a challenge [30, 34]. Kalmar et al. suggest reducing tidal volume and increasing respiratory rate and the duration of the inspiratory phase to reduce peak airway pressure [39]. An alternative is to use a pressure-controlled volume guarantee ventilation mode to deliver the tidal volume required for the lowest possible airway pressure [39].

A consequence of the upper body venous congestion caused by Trendelenburg positioning is facial and laryngeal oedema. An assessment for facial or conjunctival oedema should be performed prior to extubation and if present should alert for caution on extubating [30, 34]. A cuff leak test prior to extubating can be performed in this circumstance and if significant upper airway oedema is suspected delayed extubating may be required [30, 34, 45].

3.6 Fluid management

The intraoperative administration of intravenous (IV) fluid requires careful consideration. Excess IV fluid during Trendelenburg can exacerbate the dependent cephalad venous congestion and increase the risk of upper airway oedema, ICP and IOP [30, 34, 45]. Upper air way oedema increases the risk of post operative respiratory distress and the possible need for reintubation [30, 34, 45]. It has been suggested that total intraoperative fluids be limited to less than 2000 ml [30, 34, 45].

Intraoperative urine output is an unreliable measure of volume status with oliguria being a known effect of pneumoperitoneum [34, 45]. The mechanism may be due to reduced renal blood flow and this affect recovers on exsufflation [34, 45]. A transient rise in post operative serum creatinine may be noted but it does not cause permanent renal derangement [30, 45].

The timing of fluid administration is important, with reduced IV fluids prior to completion of the urethra-vesical anastomosis to improve vision in the surgical field. This reduces urine from the open bladder spilling into the dependent pelvic cavity [30, 34, 45]. Once the anastomosis is complete, an increase in IV fluid is desirable to mitigate against volume depletion and post operative oliguria [27, 30]. Ensuring adequate post operative urine output also serves the purpose of ensuring patency of the post operative catheter by flushing out any residual blood clot.

3.7 Neuropraxia and compartment syndromes

Mills et al. found the incidence of neuropraxia post RARP to be 7.3% in their review of 137 cases performed over 2 years [47]. Neuropraxia risk factors include operative time, time in theater, IV fluids administered and American Society of Anesthesiologists (ASA) physical status [47].

Upper limb neuropathy from RARP is often associated with techniques used to prevent the patient sliding cephalad in the Trendelenburg position. Brachial plexus injuries have been reported with the use of shoulder braces which may cause undue pressure over the acromioclavicular joint [27, 30, 31, 34]. The use of crossed chest straps has been proposed as an alternative; however this may contribute to the reduced pulmonary compliance from pneumoperitoneum [30].

We recommend avoiding shoulder braces or beanbags and utilizing a non-slip or egg crate patient mat to prevent the patient sliding cephalad in combination with wrapping of the arms by the patients' sides [30, 45]. Care needs to be taken with wrapping of the arms to prevent pressure area and ulnar neuropathy [30].

Patients undergoing RARP are at a low but serious risk of developing lower limb compartment syndrome [48]. The lower limbs have the lowest perfusion pressure due to their elevated position from lithotomy and Trendelenburg positioning [39]. Any direct compression or pressure from lithotomy stirrup positioning may exacerbate the reduced blood flow and contribute to the cascade of hypoxia and swelling [48]. Pridgeon et al. found the incidence of compartment syndrome in RARP patients to be 0.29% in their multicenter UK analysis and most of these patients required fasciotomy in treatment. They identified the patient factors of peripheral vascular disease and diabetes and peri-operative factors of patient positioning, surgeon learning curve and operative console time greater than 4 hours as risk factors [48].

Care needs to be taken to ensure the lithotomy stirrups are properly sized and positioned to ensure the supporting pressure is exerted through the heel and not the calf and that the upper calf is clear from the stirrups support [39, 46].

Lithotomy positioning and any exaggerated stretch or compression caused by the tilting into Trendelenburg position is associated with a significant risk of lower limb neuropraxia [29]. The most common lower limb neuropathies associated with lithotomy procedures are common perineal and sciatic [32]. The sciatic nerve may experience excessive stretch from over flexion of the hip and extension of the knee when placing the position into the lithotomy position [32, 49]. The common perineal nerve superficially traverses the head of fibular at the knee and therefore is susceptible to injury from direct pressure if incorrectly positioned [32, 49].

We therefore recommend due care in shifting the patient in and out of lithotomy stirrups and ensuring adequate padding particularly at the lateral leg to prevent these common nerve injuries [32].

3.8 Emergency management

Robotic radical prostatectomy carries the potential risk of intraoperative emergencies [50]. Having a well-coordinated emergency response team is essential, involving surgeons, anesthetists and operating room nurses [51–54]. Each team member should understand their designated roles and responsibilities in case of an emergency. Clarity regarding individual roles during emergencies is vital for each team member. Regular training sessions and simulated scenarios can bolster the team's readiness and ability to effectively manage critical situations.

3.8.1 Emergency undocking

Undocking the robotic system during surgery is a precise step that requires a clear understanding of potential risks. There are instances where unexpected complications prompt the surgeon to undock the robot promptly. This decision must be made cautiously, as abrupt robot withdrawal can result in bleeding, organ injury, and incomplete surgical steps. Effective communication among team members, including the anesthetists and nursing staff, is crucial to maintaining patient stability during this transition.

Undocking necessitates a thorough patient evaluation and consideration of potential conversion to open surgery. A well-defined undocking plan outlining steps for instrument withdrawal and patient positioning. Surgeons should remain aware of the situation, closely monitor vital signs, and ensure proper anesthesia management throughout the undocking process.

3.8.2 Robotic failure

In 0.2% of cases, perioperative robotic failure was observed. In one instance, the da Vinci surgical system malfunctioned during surgery, prompting the use of an alternative robot. In three other cases, intraoperative delays resulted from software failures, all of which were resolved in the operating room without any complications. Notably, no instance of robotic failure led to surgery cancelation or early anesthesia emergency [55].

3.8.3 Converting to open surgery

Switching from a minimally invasive approach to open surgery is a significant decision. Complications that cannot be managed safely using the robotic system, such as excessive bleeding or unexpected anatomical variations, often prompt this conversion [56]. Transitioning to open surgery necessitates seamless coordination, with the surgical team being well-versed in open surgical techniques, instrument handling, and patient positioning [57].

Effective communication between team members ensures a smooth transition to open surgery. Surgeons collaborate with anesthetists, nursing staff, and support personnel to facilitate an efficient shift. Adequate preoperative planning should involve discussions about scenarios that might require conversion to open surgery, along with available resources and equipment in the operating room.

3.8.4 Cardiac arrest management

Although rare, cardiac arrest can occur during RARP and demands swift and effective management. Rapid recognition and initiation of cardiopulmonary resuscitation (CPR), and immediate collaboration with the anesthesia team is crucial. Time is a crucial factor in crisis situations, and the restricted patient access inherent in robotic surgery can lead to delays in initiating effective responses. Performing undocking drills on simulators in line with well-structured emergency undocking protocols speeds up this process. These drills enhance the competence, knowledge, and confidence of the entire operating team during emergency scenarios. Integrating training sessions on emergency undocking into robotic surgery curricula is essential, ensuring that both surgeons and anesthetists are well-informed about these procedures [58].

Emergency undocking can lead to four distinct outcomes based on the underlying cause (**Figure 2**). In emergency undocking scenarios involving airway complications, cardiac arrest, bradycardia, anaphylaxis, and code red situations (fire hazards), anesthetist play a pivotal role [59].

For emergencies, the console surgeon takes charge in cases of robotic malfunction, technical issues, extensive surgical emphysema, and uncontrolled hemorrhage [60–62]. Regular simulation drills based on institutional protocols minimize patient access time (undocking time), enhance familiarity with predetermined critical actions, and boost the overall team's confidence in emergency undocking. These training sessions should take place in the actual robotic theater environment, employing the robotic patient cart alongside a mannequin or training torso. Participants' confidence, knowledge, and performance are assessed through formative simulations, followed by review sessions including lectures and reading materials [55, 63]. Summative simulations re-evaluate performance, confidence, and knowledge through multiple-choice questions and participant feedback (**Figure 3**).

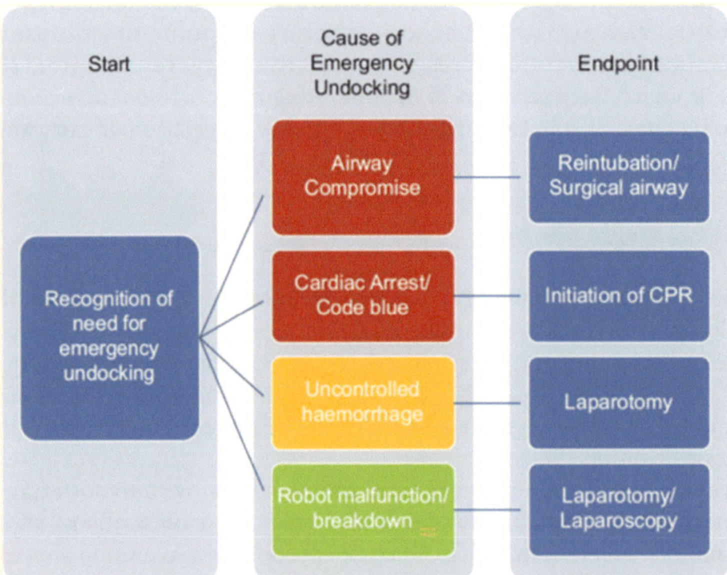

Figure 2.
The four cardinal causes and outcomes of emergency undocking. Reproduced from Shah et al. [59].

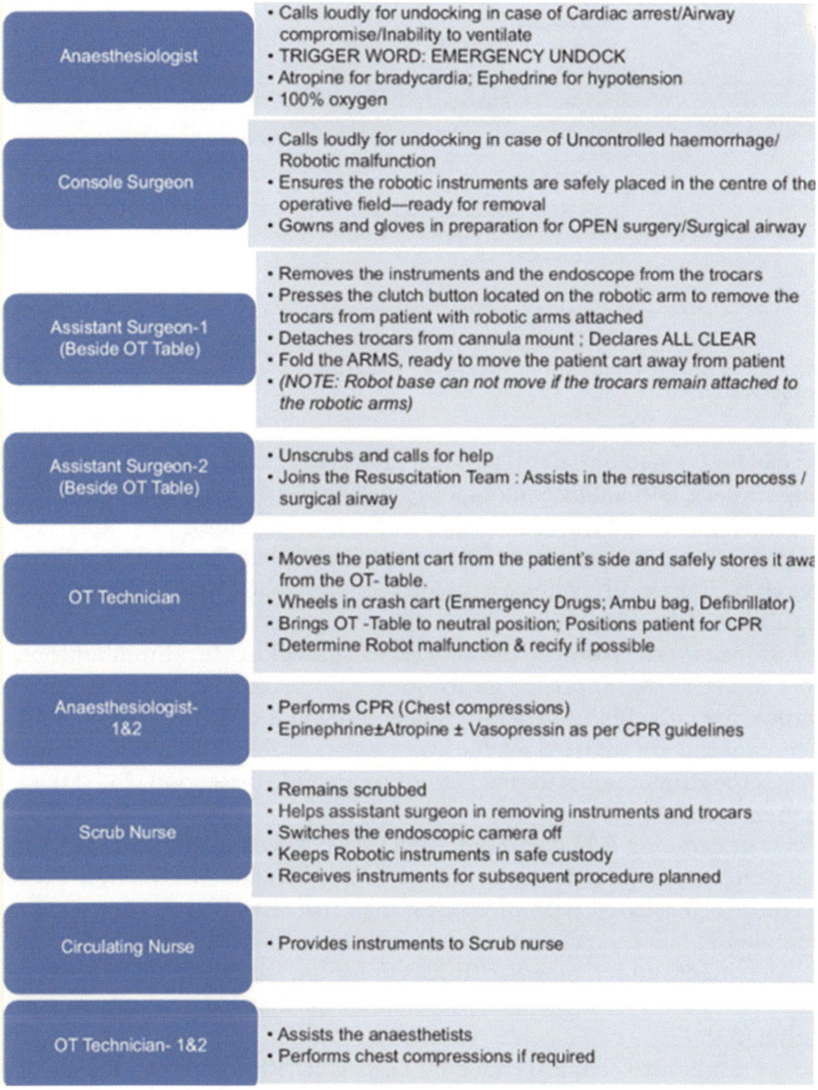

Figure 3.
Roles and responsibilities of the different members of the medical team during emergency situations in robotic surgery. Reproduced from Shah et al. [59].

4. Post operative considerations

4.1 Post operative complications

A possible, but infrequent complication following RARP is postoperative ileus which causes abdominal distention, nausea and delayed oral intake, with an occurrence rate of 1.7%. For most patients, conservative management with intravenous fluids and bowel rest suffice, while a small subset require gastric decompression using a nasogastric tube. More serious early post-operative complications that may require further surgical intervention, include bowel injury, port site hernias, intrabdominal bleeding, and anastomotic disruption. All these complications are exceedingly

Risk group	Risk factors	Likelihood of VTE
Low	—	1X
Medium	One of the following: • age ≥ 75 years • BMI ≥35 • VTE in a 1st degree relative	2X
High	• Previous VTE • ≥ 2 of the above risk factors	4X

Table 4.
Venous thromboembolism risk stratification. Reproduced and adapted from the EAU guidelines for thromboprophylaxis [67].

rare and can be avoided by careful surgical dissection at the time of RARP. Anemia following surgery, defined by hemoglobin levels below 10 g dL, is found in 1.0% of cases, leading to blood transfusions. Postoperative pulmonary emboli occur in 0.2% of patients and are prevented by appropriate venous thromboembolism (VTE) prophylaxis including calf compressors intra-operatively, TEDS and prophylactic anticoagulation [64–66].

The European Association of Urology (EAU) guidelines for thromboprophylaxis suggests a risk stratified approach for the prescription of extended prophylaxis for 4 weeks post operatively (**Table 4**) [67]. Recommendations are specific to radical prostatectomy and are adjusted for the lower risk post RARP compared to open and for whether the patient underwent a pelvic lymph node dissection (PLND) which confers greater risk.

Patients undergoing RARP without PLND are not recommended for pharmacological prophylaxis. Patients undergoing RARP with standard PLND are recommended for pharmacological prophylaxis if high risk only. Patients undergoing RARP with extended PLND are recommended for pharmacological prophylaxis if medium or high. All patients undergoing RARP, except for low-risk patient undergoing RARP without PLND, have a weak recommendation for mechanical prophylaxis until ambulation [67].

A recent randomized clinical trial on VTE post RARP comparing mechanical prophylaxis with pharmacological prophylaxis during admission demonstrates contemporary experience of VTE post RARP [68]. The rate of overall VTE at 30 days was 2.8% with pharmacological prophylaxis and 2.9% without [68]. All VTE episodes occurred in patients who underwent PLND [68]. There was no increase in symptomatic lymphocele, bleeding or other complications with the use of pharmacological VTE prophylaxis [68].

4.2 Enhanced recovery after surgery

The implementation of Enhanced Recovery After Surgery (ERAS) protocols has revolutionized postoperative care following robotic prostatectomy, offering a comprehensive approach to improving patient outcomes and recovery. ERAS protocols are designed to streamline perioperative care, reduce complications, and accelerate patient recovery through evidence-based practices. In the context of robotic prostatectomy, the integration of ERAS protocols holds significant promise.

ERAS protocols following robotic prostatectomy encompass a range of interventions that span the preoperative, intraoperative, and postoperative phases [59–62]. Preoperative elements often involve patient education, nutritional optimization, and the reduction of preoperative fasting period. These measures not only enhance patient understanding but also contribute to improved physical condition, better immune function, and overall preparedness for surgery. Intraoperatively, strategies such as minimal invasive techniques, judicious fluid management, and opioid-sparing anesthesia aim to minimize the physiological stress of surgery, reducing the risk of complications and expediting postoperative recovery [55, 61, 63, 69–71].

One of the key advantages of ERAS protocols in the postoperative phase is the early initiation of oral intake, which aids in maintaining gut motility, reducing the chance of postoperative ileus, and hence reducing the duration of hospitalization. Pain management techniques that prioritize multimodal analgesia over opioids mitigate side effects and enhance patient comfort while facilitating earlier ambulation and mobilization.

Additionally, ERAS protocols emphasize the importance of early ambulation, which promotes respiratory function, prevents thromboembolic events, and contributes to faster recovery. Lastly, ERAS protocol in certain institutions mandates drain removal if output is <50 ml in a 24 hours' period on day 1 post-operatively. This significantly reduces patient's length of stay [64–66, 72, 73].

The implementation of ERAS protocols also addresses patient-specific factors, tailoring interventions to individual needs. This personalized approach not only improves patient satisfaction but also potentially reduces the length of hospital stay and associated costs. Furthermore, ERAS protocols emphasize the role of a multidisciplinary team, promoting effective communication among surgeons, anesthetists, nurses, and other healthcare professionals. This collaboration ensures the smooth execution of the various components of the protocol, minimizing variability in care delivery [74].

ERAS protocols have optimized recovery following robotic prostatectomy. By focusing on evidence-based practices that encompass the entire perioperative continuum, ERAS protocols enhance patient outcomes, decrease complications, and expedite recovery.

4.3 Functional rehabilitation

Pelvic floor exercises and penile rehabilitation have emerged as vital components of the comprehensive postoperative care strategy following robotic prostatectomy. This discussion underscores their significance in enhancing the quality of life and restoring sexual function in patients who have undergone this procedure.

Pelvic floor exercises, often referred to as Kegel exercises, target the muscles that support the bladder, prostate, and rectum. They have gained prominence as a non-invasive and effective approach to addressing postoperative urinary incontinence, a common concern after prostate surgery [56–59, 75]. By strengthening the pelvic floor muscles, these exercises contribute to improved urinary control and minimize the extent of incontinence. Encouraging patients to engage in these exercises preoperatively and postoperatively empowers them to actively participate in their recovery journey and regain continence more swiftly [58].

Equally crucial in the realm of postoperative recovery is penile rehabilitation, which focuses on maintaining erectile function following robotic prostatectomy. The disruption of neurovascular bundles during surgery can lead to temporary or prolonged erectile dysfunction [56]. Penile rehabilitation strategies encompass a range of interventions, including pharmacological agents, vacuum erection devices, and intracavernosal injections, all of which aim to prevent the irreversible loss of penile tissue and promote vascular health. Additionally, early engagement in sexual activity and counseling play pivotal roles in facilitating psychological adaptation and optimizing sexual outcomes [75].

The integration of both pelvic floor exercises and penile rehabilitation into the postoperative care plan acknowledges the multidimensional nature of recovery after robotic prostatectomy. While these interventions primarily address specific functional concerns, they also extend their benefits to psychological well-being and overall quality of life [64, 65, 70–73]. By actively involving patients in their recovery process and offering tailored solutions, healthcare providers empower individuals to take ownership of their sexual health and urinary continence.

However, successful implementation of pelvic floor exercises and penile rehabilitation necessitates patient education and adherence. Healthcare professionals play a pivotal role in imparting the significance of these interventions and providing guidance on their correct execution. Collaborative efforts between urologists, physical therapists, and sexual health specialists ensure that patients receive comprehensive support throughout their recovery journey [66, 74].

In conclusion, pelvic floor exercises and penile rehabilitation represent integral pillars of the postoperative care regimen for patients undergoing robotic prostatectomy. By addressing urinary incontinence and erectile dysfunction, respectively, these interventions contribute to improved functional outcomes and enhance the overall quality of life. The comprehensive approach to recovery that includes both physical exercises and sexual rehabilitation underscores the holistic nature of care and reflects the commitment to restoring patients' well-being in its entirety.

5. Concluding remarks

As RARP is increasingly adopted as the surgical modality of choice for localized prostate cancer, a thorough understanding of its implications for successful perioperative care is imperative. Patient selection, pre-operative optimization and patient education are critical to prepare for success. A thorough understanding of the anesthetic and physiological implications of Trendelenburg position, lithotomy and pneumoperitoneum in combination with robotic docking is necessary for successful intraoperative management and emergency management should the need arise. Finally, attention to the principles of enhanced recovery after surgery and the specifics of post operative care following RARP is critical to maximizing patient outcomes.

Author details

Amandeep Virk[1,2], Victor Yu[2], Wenjie Zhong[3,4], Samuel Davies[2] and Scott Leslie[1,2,3,5]*

1 Department of Uro-Oncology, Chris O'Brien Lifehouse, Camperdown, NSW, Australia

2 Department of Urology, Royal Prince Alfred Hospital, Camperdown, NSW, Australia

3 The University of Sydney, Camperdown, NSW, Australia

4 The University of New South Wales, Kensington, NSW, Australia

5 The Institute of Academic Surgery at Royal Prince Alfred Hospital, Sydney, Australia

*Address all correspondence to: scottleslie@me.com

References

[1] Culp MB, Soerjomataram I, Efstathiou JA, Bray F, Jemal A. Recent global patterns in prostate cancer incidence and mortality rates. European Urology. 2020;**77**(1):38-52

[2] Yaxley JW, Coughlin GD, Chambers SK, Occhipinti S, Samaratunga H, Zajdlewicz L, et al. Robot-assistedlaparoscopicprostatectomy versus open radical retropubic prostatectomy: Early outcomes from a randomised controlled phase 3 study. Lancet. 2016;**388**(10049):1057-1066

[3] Coughlin GD, Yaxley JW, Chambers SK, Occhipinti S, Samaratunga H, Zajdlewicz L, et al. Robot-assisted laparoscopic prostatectomy versus open radical retropubic prostatectomy: 24-month outcomes from a randomised controlled study. The Lancet Oncology. 2018;**19**(8):1051-1060

[4] Korc-Grodzicki B, Root JC, Alici Y. Prevention of post-operative delirium in older patients with cancer undergoing surgery. Journal of Geriatric Oncology. 2015;**6**(1):60-69

[5] McIsaac DI, Taljaard M, Bryson GL, Beaulé PE, Gagné S, Hamilton G, et al. Frailty as a predictor of death or new disability after surgery: A prospective cohort study. Annals of Surgery. 2020;**271**(2):283-289

[6] Ethun CG, Bilen MA, Jani AB, Maithel SK, Ogan K, Master VA. Frailty and cancer: Implications for oncology surgery, medical oncology, and radiation oncology. CA: A Cancer Journal for Clinicians. 2017;**67**(5):362-377

[7] Mottet N, van den Bergh RCN, Briers E, Van den Broeck T, Cumberbatch MG, De Santis M, et al. EAU-EANM-ESTRO-ESUR-SIOG guidelines on prostate cancer-2020 update. Part 1: Screening, diagnosis, and local treatment with curative intent. European Urology. 2021;**79**(2):243-262

[8] Blezien O, Bentellis I, Tibi B, Shaikh A, Rambaud C, Boulahssass R, et al. Robot assisted radical prostatectomy in fit older patients compared to a standard population: Clinical characteristics, surgical, oncological and functional outcomes. Progrès en Urologie. 2023;**33**(5):272-278

[9] Xia Z, Fu X, Li J, Yuan X, Wu J, Tang L. Application of robot-assisted radical prostatectomy in men over 75 years: An analysis of comparative outcomes. The Aging Male. 2023;**26**(1):2166919

[10] Kumar S, Shelley M, Harrison C, Coles B, Wilt TJ, Mason MD. Neo-adjuvant and adjuvant hormone therapy for localised and locally advanced prostate cancer. Cochrane Database of Systematic Reviews. 2006;**2006**(4):Cd006019

[11] Liu W, Yao Y, Liu X, Liu Y, Zhang GM. Neoadjuvant hormone therapy for patients with high-risk prostate cancer: A systematic review and meta-analysis. Asian Journal of Andrology. 2021;**23**(4):429-436

[12] Yanagisawa T, Rajwa P, Quhal F, et al. Neoadjuvant androgen receptor signaling inhibitors before radical prostatectomy for non-metastatic advanced prostate cancer: A systematic review. Journal of Personalized Medicine. 2023;**13**(4):641

[13] Fleisher LA, Fleischmann KE, Auerbach AD, Barnason SA, Beckman JA,

Bozkurt B, et al. 2014 ACC/AHA guideline on perioperative cardiovascular evaluation and management of patients undergoing noncardiac surgery: Executive summary: A report of the American College of Cardiology/ American Heart Association Task Force on Practice Guidelines. Circulation. 2014;**130**(24):2215-2245

[14] Awad H, Walker CM, Shaikh M, Dimitrova GT, Abaza R, O'Hara J. Anesthetic considerations for robotic prostatectomy: A review of the literature. Journal of Clinical Anesthesia. 2012;**24**(6):494-504

[15] Awad H, Santilli S, Ohr M, Roth A, Yan W, Fernandez S, et al. The effects of steep trendelenburg positioning on intraocular pressure during robotic radical prostatectomy. Anesthesia and Analgesia. 2009;**109**(2):473-478

[16] Han H, Cao Z, Qin Y, Wei X, Ruan Y, Cao Y, et al. Morbid obesity is adversely associated with perioperative outcomes in patients undergoing robot-assisted laparoscopic radical prostatectomy. Canadian Urological Association Journal. 2020;**14**(11):E574-Ee81

[17] OPTIFAST. Shop by Diet Plans/ Intensive Level. Available from: https:// www.optifast.com.au/diet-plans/ intensive-level.list [Accessed: September 15, 2023]

[18] Wilding JPH, Batterham RL, Calanna S, et al. Once-weekly Semaglutide in adults with overweight or obesity. The New England Journal of Medicine. 2021;**384**(11):989-1002

[19] Leslie S, Jackson S, Broe M, van Diepen DC, Stanislaus C, Steffens D, et al. Improved early and late continence following robot-assisted radical prostatectomy with concurrent bladder neck fascial sling (RoboSling). BJUI Compass. 2023;**4**(5):597-604

[20] Spinelli MG, Cozzi G, Grasso A, Talso M, Varisco D, Abed El Rahman D, et al. Ralp and Rocco stitch: Original technique. Urologia. 2011;**78**(Suppl 18):35-38

[21] Chang JI, Lam V, Patel MI. Preoperative pelvic floor muscle exercise and postprostatectomy incontinence: A systematic review and meta-analysis. European Urology. 2016;**69**(3):460-467

[22] Kretschmer A, Buchner A, Grabbert M, Sommer A, Herlemann A, Stief CG, et al. Perioperative patient education improves long-term satisfaction rates of low-risk prostate cancer patients after radical prostatectomy. World Journal of Urology. 2017;**35**(8):1205-1212

[23] Wake N, Rosenkrantz AB, Huang R, Park KU, Wysock JS, Taneja SS, et al. Patient-specific 3D printed and augmented reality kidney and prostate cancer models: Impact on patient education. 3D Printing in Medicine. 2019;**5**(1):4

[24] Gyomber D, Lawrentschuk N, Wong P, Parker F, Bolton DM. Improving informed consent for patients undergoing radical prostatectomy using multimedia techniques: A prospective randomized crossover study. BJU International. 2010;**106**(8):1152-1156

[25] Clinical Excellence Commission. Guidelines on Perioperative Management of Anticoagulant and Antiplatelet Agents. Sydney: Clinical Excellence Commission; 2018

[26] Yee DS, Ornstein DK. Repair of rectal injury during robotic-assisted laparoscopic prostatectomy. Urology. 2008;**72**(2):428-431

[27] Hsu RL, Kaye AD, Urman RD. Anesthetic challenges in robotic-assisted urologic surgery. Revista de Urología. 2013;**15**(4):178-184

[28] Lee JR. Anesthetic considerations for robotic surgery. Korean Journal of Anesthesiology. 2014;**66**(1):3-11. DOI: 10.4097/kjae.2014.66.1.3

[29] Wayne G, Wei J, Atri E, et al. Trends in positioning for robotic prostatectomy: Results from a survey of the endourological society. Cureus. 2021;**13**(1):e12628. Published 2021 Jan 11

[30] Gainsburg DM. Anesthetic concerns for robotic-assisted laparoscopic radical prostatectomy. Minerva Anestesiologica. 2012;**78**(5):596-604

[31] Chitlik A. Safe positioning for robotic-assisted laparoscopic prostatectomy. AORN Journal. 2011;**94**(1):37-48

[32] Tollefson MK, Boorjian SA, Leibovich BC. Chapter 20 - Complications of the Incision and Patient Positioning, Complications of Urologic Surgery. 4th ed. Philadelphia, USA: W.B. Saunders; 2010. pp. 225-236. ISBN: 9781416045724

[33] Armstrong M, Moore RA. Anatomy, patient positioning [updated 2022 Oct 31]. In: StatPearls [Internet]. Treasure Island (FL): StatPearls Publishing; 2023. Available from: https://www.ncbi.nlm.nih.gov/books/NBK513320/

[34] Pathirana S, Kam P. Anaesthetic issues in robotic-assisted minimally invasive surgery. Anaesthesia and Intensive Care. 2018;**46**(1):25-35

[35] Ripa M, Schipa C, Kopsacheilis N, et al. The impact of steep trendelenburg position on intraocular pressure. Journal of Clinical Medicine. 2022;**11**(10):2844. Published 2022 May 18

[36] Sampat A, Parakati I, Kunnavakkam R, et al. Corneal abrasion in hysterectomy and prostatectomy: Role of laparoscopic and robotic assistance. Anesthesiology. 2015;**122**(5):994-1001

[37] Danic MJ, Chow M, Alexander G, Bhandari A, Menon M, Brown M. Anesthesia considerations for robotic-assisted laparoscopic prostatectomy: A review of 1,500 cases. Journal of Robotic Surgery. 2007;**1**(2):119-123

[38] Segal KL, Fleischut PM, Kim C, et al. Evaluation and treatment of perioperative corneal abrasions. Journal of Ophthalmology. 2014;**2014**:901901

[39] Kalmar A, De Wolf A, Hendrickx J. Anesthetic considerations for robotic surgery in the steep Trendelenburg position. Advances in Anesthesia. 2012;**30**(1):75-96

[40] Wiesinger C, Schoeb DS, Stockhammer M, et al. Cerebral oxygenation in 45-degree trendelenburg position for robot-assisted radical prostatectomy: A single-center, open, controlled pilot study. BMC Urology. 2020;**20**(1):198

[41] Nishikawa M, Watanabe H, Kurahashi T. Effects of 25- and 30-degree Trendelenburg positions on intraocular pressure changes during robot-assisted radical prostatectomy. Prostate International. 2017;**5**(4):135-138

[42] Raz O, Boesel TW, Arianayagam M, et al. The effect of the modified Z trendelenburg position on intraocular pressure during robotic assisted laparoscopic radical prostatectomy: A randomized, controlled

study. The Journal of Urology. 2015;**193**(4):1213-1219

[43] Neudecker J, Sauerland S, Neugebauer E, et al. The European Association for Endoscopic Surgery clinical practice guideline on the pneumoperitoneum for laparoscopic surgery. Surgical Endoscopy. 2002;**16**(7):1121-1143

[44] Lestar M, Gunnarsson L, Lagerstrand L, Wiklund P, Odeberg-Wernerman S. Hemodynamic perturbations during robot-assisted laparoscopic radical prostatectomy in 45° Trendelenburg position. Anesthesia and Analgesia. 2011;**113**(5):1069-1075

[45] Baltayian S. A brief review: Anesthesia for robotic prostatectomy. Journal of Robotic Surgery. 2008;**2**(2):59

[46] Chang CH, Lee HK, Nam SH. The displacement of the tracheal tube during robot-assisted radical prostatectomy. European Journal of Anaesthesiology. 2010;**27**(5):478-480

[47] Mills JT, Burris MB, Warburton DJ, Conaway MR, Schenkman NS, Krupski TL. Positioning injuries associated with robotic assisted urological surgery. The Journal of Urology. 2013;**190**(2):580-584

[48] Pridgeon S, Bishop CV, Adshead J. Lower limb compartment syndrome as a complication of robot-assisted radical prostatectomy: The UK experience. BJU International. 2013;**112**(4):485-488

[49] Cestari A, Ferrari M, Zanoni M, et al. Side docking of the da Vinci robotic system for radical prostatectomy: Advantages over traditional docking. Journal of Robotic Surgery. 2015;**9**(3):243-247

[50] Coelho R, Palmer K, Rocco B, Moniz R, Chauhan S, Orvieto M, et al. Early complication rates in a single-surgeon series of 2500 robotic-assisted radical prostatectomies: Report applying a standardized grading. European Urology. 2010;**57**:945-952

[51] Dall'Oglio M, Srougi M, Pereira D, Nesrallah A, Andreoni C, Kauffmann J, et al. Rupture of vesicourethral anastomosis following radical retropubic prostatectomy. International Brazilian Journal of Urology. 2003;**29**:221-227

[52] Dindo D, Demartines N, Clavien P. Classification of surgical complications: A new proposal with evaluation in a cohort of 6336 patients and results of a survey. Surgery. 2004;**240**:205-213

[53] Gill I, Kavoussi L, Clayman R, Ehrlich R, Evans R, Fuchs G, et al. Complications of laparoscopic nephrectomy in 185 patients: A multi-institutional review. The Journal of Urology. 1995;**154**:479-483

[54] Gill I, Ukimura O, Rubinstein M, Finelli A, Moinzadeh A, Singh D, et al. Lateral pedicle control during laparoscopic radical prostatectomy: Refined technique. Urology. 2005;**65**:23-27

[55] Patel V, Palmer K, Coughlin G, Samavedi S. Robot-assisted laparoscopic radical prostatectomy: Perioperative outcomes of 1500 cases. Journal of Endourology. 2008;**22**:2299-2305

[56] Keegan K, Cookson M. Complications of pelvic lymph node dissection for prostate cancer. Current Urology Reports. 2011;**12**:203-208

[57] Larobina M, Nottle P. Complete evidence regarding major vascular injuries during laparoscopic access. Surgical Laparoscopy, Endoscopy

& Percutaneous Techniques. 2005;**15**:119-123

[58] Lebeau T, Rouprêt M, Ferhi K, Chartier-Kastler E, Richard F, Bitker M, et al. Assessing the complications of laparoscopic robot-assisted surgery: The case of radical prostatectomy. A modified Clavien–Dindo classification also was used to account for intraoperative complications. Surgical Endoscopy. 2011;**25**:536-542

[59] Shah SB, Chawla R, Rawal SK. Rapid undocking protocol for the da Vinci surgical robot during emergency situations. Indian Journal of Anaesthesia. 2023;**67**(4):398-400

[60] Lowrance W, Eastham J, Savage C, Maschino A, Laudone V, Dechet C, et al. Contemporary open and robotic radical prostatectomy practice patterns among urologists in the United States. The Journal of Urology. 2012;**187**:2087-2092

[61] Merlin T, Hiller J, Maddern G, Jamieson G, Brown A, Kolbe A. Systematic review of the safety and effectiveness of methods used to establish pneumoperitoneum in laparoscopic surgery. The British Journal of Surgery. 2003;**90**:668-669

[62] Nguyen M, Turna B, Santos B, Frota R, Aron M, Stein R, et al. The use of an endoscopic stapler versus suture ligature for dorsal vein control in laparoscopic prostatectomy: Operative outcomes. BJU International. 2008;**101**:463-466

[63] Ovroutski S, Ewert P, Schubel J, Lange P, Hetzer R. A rare complication of laparoscopic surgery: Iatrogenic arteriovenous fistula with high-output cardiac failure. Surgical Laparoscopy, Endoscopy & Percutaneous Techniques. 2001;**11**:334-337

[64] Stolzenburg J, Rabenalt R, Do M, Lee B, Truss N, McNeill A, et al. Complications of endoscopic extraperitoneal radical prostatectomy (EERPE): Prevention and management. World Journal of Urology. 2006;**24**:668-675

[65] Stolzenburg J, Truss M. Technique of laparoscopic (endoscopic) radical prostatectomy. BJU International. 2003;**91**:749-757

[66] Tewari A, Sooriakumaran P, Bloch D, Seshadri-Kreaden U, Hebert A, Wiklund P. Positive surgical margin and perioperative complication rates of primary surgical treatments for prostate cancer: A systematic review and meta-analysis comparing retropubic, laparoscopic, and robotic prostatectomy. European Urology. 2012;**62**:1-15

[67] Tikkinen KAO, Cartwright R, Gould MK, Naspro R, Novara G, Sandset PM, et al. Thromboprophylaxis Guideline Panel. EAU Guidelines on Thromboprophylaxis in Urological Surgery. Arnhem, The Netherlands: EAU Guidelines Office; 2017. Available from: http://uroweb.org/guidelines/compilations-of-all-guidelines/ [Accessed: September 15, 2023]

[68] Patel HD, Faisal FA, Trock BJ, et al. Effect of pharmacologic prophylaxis on venous thromboembolism after radical prostatectomy: The PREVENTER randomized clinical trial. European Urology. 2020;**78**(3):360-368

[69] Novara G, Ficarra V, Rosen R, Artibani W, Costello A, Eastham J, et al. Systematic review and meta-analysis of perioperative outcomes and complications after robot-assisted radical prostatectomy. European Urology. 2012;**62**:431-452

[70] Pereira AJ, Gamarra QM, Leibar TA, Astobieta Odriozola A,

Ibarluzea González G. Incidencias y complicaciones en nuestras primeras 250 prostatectomias radicales roboticas. Actas Urologicas Españolas. 2010;**34**:428-439

[71] Shekarriz B, Upadhyay J, Wood D. Intraoperative, perioperative, and long-term complications of radical prostatectomy. The Urologic Clinics of North America. 2001;**28**:639-653

[72] Siqueira T, Kuo R, Gardner T, Paterson R, Stevens L, Lingeman J, et al. Major complications in 213 laparoscopic nephrectomy cases: The Indianapolis experience. The Journal of Urology. 2002;**168**:1361-1365

[73] Stolzenburg J, Do M, Rabenalt R, Dietel A, Pfeiffer H, Reinhardt F, et al. Endoscopic extraperitoneal radical prostatectomy. In: Stolzenburg J, Türk I, Liatsikos E, editors. Laparoscopic and Robot-Assisted Surgery in Urology. Berlin: Springer; 2007. pp. 121-133

[74] Zorn K, Katz M, Bernstein A, Shikanov S, Brendler C, Zagaja Z, et al. Laparoscopy and robotics pelvic lymphadenectomy during robot-assisted radical prostatectomy: Assessing nodal yield, perioperative outcomes, and complications. Urology. 2009;**74**:296-302

[75] Lasser M, Renzulli J II, Turini G III, Haleblian G, Sax H, Pareek G. An unbiased prospective report of perioperative complications of robot-assisted laparoscopic radical prostatectomy. Urology. 2010;**75**:1083-1089

Chapter 5

Perspective Chapter: Perioperative Management in Cardiac Surgery

Maria del Carmen Renteria Arellano
and Hugo de Jesus Ballesteros Loyo

Abstract

The patient undergoing heart surgery must be managed differently and more intensively than the average surgical patient. These are patients with important hereditary and pathological antecedents as well as co-morbidities and chronic pathologies. For this reason, studies and compilations have been carried out in order to improve the conditions of the patients and to have a favourable evolution. Likewise, advances in technology, as well as pharmacological advances have brought new strategies for the improvement of these patients, mainly by undergoing cardiopulmonary bypass. This chapter is intended to be a guide for intensivists and the best management of patients undergoing cardiac surgery.

Keywords: cardiopulmonary bypass (CPB), preoperative medicine, cardiovascular surgery, intensive care medicine, intra-aortic balloon pump (IABP)

1. Introduction

Cardiac surgery, when properly indicated, saves lives almost immediately. However, it is rarely performed in a timely manner or as a last resort in patients with significant cardiac damage.

In recent years, it has progressed exponentially, creating new expectations for patients with heart disease to recover quickly and without complications.

Different groups and/or associations have been created, such as the ERAS (Enhanced Recovery After Surgery) programme which presents a transdisciplinary enhanced care initiative to promote the recovery of patients undergoing surgery throughout their perioperative journey [1].

These programmes aim to reduce complications and promote an earlier return to normal activities for patients [2, 3]. The ERAS protocol has been associated with a reduction in all complications and length of in-hospital stay of up to 50% compared to conventional perioperative management of the non-cardiac surgery patient [4–6].

Cardiac surgery covers a wide range of surgical techniques and a variety of physiological insults that can have an impact on postoperative recovery. As in any other speciality, the patient has his or her own pre-existing comorbidities which have a major effect on the outcome. These factors range from pre-existing medical conditions to the patient's cognitive ability or nutritional status prior to surgery.

 IntechOpen

2. Perioperative medicine

This is a new and growing area of medicine that is of great interest in the surgical world, as it includes different specialities, in this case, cardiology, critical care medicine, anaesthesiology and cardiac surgery.

It is mainly supported by evidence-based medicine, and, as previously mentioned, by groups and/or protocols such as ERAS, which have allowed to involve patients in their care, reduce the stress response to surgical trauma and allow the patient to regain normal function more quickly after major surgery.

In recent years, cardiovascular surgery has evolved by leaps and bounds with several advances including improved myocardial protection, safer systemic perfusion during extracorporeal circulation (ECC) and cerebral protection in situations of circulatory arrest (which can occur for multiple causes, and is primarily the surgeon's decision), as well as the implementation of safe surgery protocols during surgery; standard monitoring supported by transesophageal echocardiography of technical complications; the incorporation of minimally invasive surgical techniques, the implantation of transcatheter valves without sutures and the development of multimodal rehabilitation among many others. The aim is to improve the patient's quality of life and return to normal life as soon as possible and with as little morbidity as possible [7].

As in all surgery, health personnel try to keep the perioperative period as short as possible, and this does not exclude cardiac surgery [8].

The perioperative period is defined as: The entire surgical process, whether urgent or scheduled, that a patient undergoes, comprising the following phases:

- Preoperative: From the moment the patient is informed that a surgical intervention is required until his or her arrival in the operating theatre. It includes the anamnesis in the different assessments, complementary tests and pre-surgical preparation.

- Intraoperative: Covers from the time the patient enters the operating theatre until he/she leaves.

- Postoperative: It covers three periods:

    a. The immediate postoperative period: From the end of the surgical procedure until recovery from the effects of anaesthesia. It usually takes place in the post post-anaesthesia recovery room; in the case of cardiac surgery, it is generally in the intensive care unit. It can last between 24 and 72 hours.

    b. The mediate postoperative period: This includes recovery from the effects of anaesthesia to recovery in hospitalisation units.

    c. The late postoperative period: Includes the patient's recovery at home until reintegration into normal life. It is considered more of an epidemiological concept.

3. Preoperative period in cardiac surgery

3.1 Preoperative preparation

The patient should be the focus of attention [9, 10]. This implies that the physician must provide the patient with all the necessary information to obtain informed consent for surgery, as well as a detailed description of possible events and/or complications, the importance of preoperative interventions for the surgery to go well and the expectations for the postoperative period (which are mainly the improvement of the quality of life).

Generally, the definitive diagnosis is made by the clinical and/or interventional cardiologist, who must explain all the appropriate treatments according to the condition, and according to his or her experience and knowledge of medical advances, which would be ideal for the pathology to be treated.

On the other hand, the cardiologist should also be the doctor who identifies and/or manages the patient's pre-existing diseases, such as systemic arterial hypertension, diabetes mellitus, arrhythmias, nutritional status, psychological status, anaemia, renal insufficiency, etc. However, nowadays with specialised medicine, it is preferred that it be managed by an internist or with the subspecialty that corresponds to the diagnosis.

Likewise, the treating physician must insist on changes in hygienic-dietary habits (such as giving up alcohol, smoking and drug addiction) and improving cardiopulmonary fitness [11].

3.2 Risk assessment and risk stratification

All patients undergoing cardiac surgery should be assessed for intraoperative risk. There are several scores that assess this risk, such as the EuroSCORE (European System for Cardiac Operative Risk Evaluation) or the STS (Society of Thoracic Surgeons) surgical risk. This information provides greater understanding for the patient, improves decision making, allows preoperative optimisation and enables modification of the surgical technique or procedure if necessary.

3.3 Pre-rehabilitation

It is the process of increasing the patient's functional status and ability to cope with stress after surgery.

This includes education, correction of nutritional deficiencies, improvement of physical fitness and psychological and social support. The goal of these interventions is to reduce the patient's anxiety, improve muscle quality and, in the background, to check that the patient has a full understanding of the surgical process, or to insist on its explanation. This stage includes:

a. Education in cardiac surgery: This should be carried out as an individual course and teach what the surgery is based on, surgical techniques, etc., and in this way reduce and clarify doubts that the patient and/or relatives have, and, secondarily, reduce the patients' stress. These sessions emphasise the importance of being active, living well, eating well and exercising or training to improve respiratory and muscular function before surgery.

b. Preoperative exercise: Safe exercise programmes are available for patients with cardiorespiratory impairment, which if performed regularly improve physical and mental fitness, as it can increase the ratio of lean body mass to body fat. It also helps (although not in all patients) to decrease perioperative sympathetic dysregulation and insulin resistance [12]. Additional benefits are on the patient's physical and psychological preparation for surgery, which helps to reduce postoperative complications, decrease the length of hospital stay and the patient has an adequate recovery before returning home [13]. This, of course, should be individualised according to each patient's health status.

c. Lifestyle modifications: It is common knowledge that excesses contribute to the progressive deterioration of patients, thus smoking, excessive alcohol consumption and obesity are associated with perioperative complications and poorer surgical outcomes. They can lead to serious complications, including wound infections, and only small changes in daily life, such as smoking cessation and weight loss, can significantly reduce them [14].

3.4 Minimising fasting and preoperative carbohydrate loading

Although not always accepted, mainly by anaesthesiologists, it has been shown to be safe to give clear fluids up to 2 hours before induction of anaesthesia. Several studies mention that giving the patient a carbohydrate drink (usually with 24 g of complex carbohydrates) 2 hours before surgery is a mainstay of preoperative management and is supported by most ERAS programmes. This measure is sufficiently adequate as it is associated with a reduction in insulin resistance and tissue glycosylation, stabilisation of postoperative glucose concentration and an earlier return of normal gastrointestinal function. Articles have already established that administering carbohydrate beverages prior to cardiac surgery is safe and improves cardiac function immediately after Cardiopulmonary bypass (CPB) [15].

3.5 Preoperative strategies

a. Preoperative measurement of haemoglobin A1c for risk stratification: This simple test should be performed in practically all patients with any diagnosis. And in patients who will undergo surgery, all the more so, in order to establish optimal preoperative glycaemic control. Ideally, patients should maintain a haemoglobin A1c level of less than 6.5%; this has been associated with a significant decrease in sternal and/or mediastinal wound infections, ischaemic events and other complications [16, 17]. If the HbAc1 level is higher than 7%, significant dysglycaemia can occur, which is difficult to manage in the immediate postoperative period [18].

b. Preoperative albumin measurement for risk stratification: It is widely known that low preoperative serum albumin in patients undergoing surgery is associated with an increased risk of morbidity and mortality after surgery. Hypoalbuminaemia is a perioperative prognostic risk factor, correlating with longer mechanical ventilation time, acute kidney injury (AKI), infections, longer hospital stay and mortality. Correction of serum albumin prior to surgery is necessary to avoid these comorbidities [19–21].

c. Preoperative correction of nutritional deficiency: It would be great if all surgical patients were well nourished, however, this is not common. For malnourished patients, oral nutritional supplements can be given, but only have an effect if given 10 days prior to surgery. This improvement is associated with reduced prevalence of infection and improved healing. However, there is not yet a well-established programme for improving nutritional status [9, 10].

3.6 Intraoperative period

This period is characterised by the intervention of the surgeon and his skill, but just as importantly by the anaesthetic management as well as the management of the ECC by the perfusionist. However, each of these players has their own protocols depending on the type of surgery at the time and the likely complications or incidents during this period.

It should be remembered that the open heart patient requires specialised care because ECC alters physiological systems (**Figures 1** and **2**).

CPB (**Figures 3** and **4**) produces a generalised inflammatory response caused by the contact of blood with the synthetic surfaces of the bypass circuit [22]. This inflammatory response results in a series of complex reactions that activate the complement, coagulation and fibrinolytic cascade, leading to bleeding, microemboli, fluid retention and an altered hormonal response [23–25].

ECC is a non-specific activator of the inflammatory system. Once ECC is discontinued, widespread complement activation occurs with elevations of anaphylatoxins C3a and C5a and this activation may result in pulmonary leukocyte sequestration and superoxide production and then further increasing leukocyte activation and

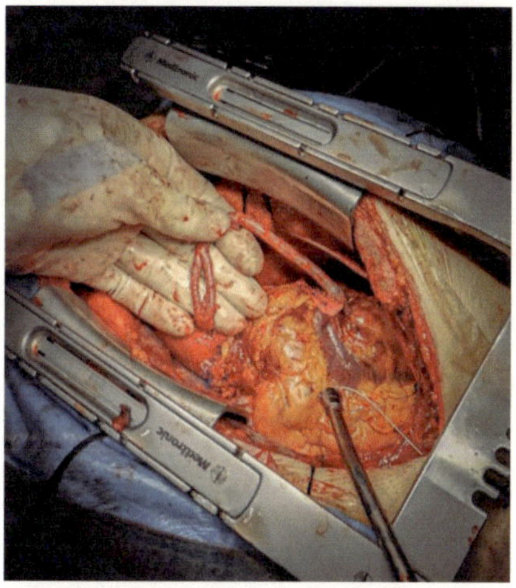

Figure 1.
Open heart surgery: Aortocoronary revascularization.

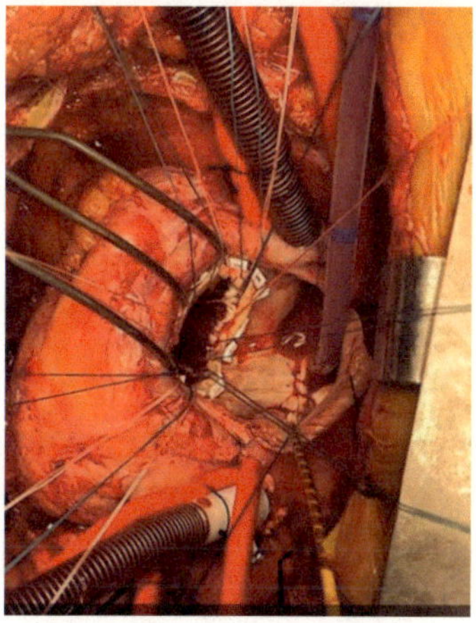

Figure 2.
Open heart surgery: Placement of valve prosthesis.

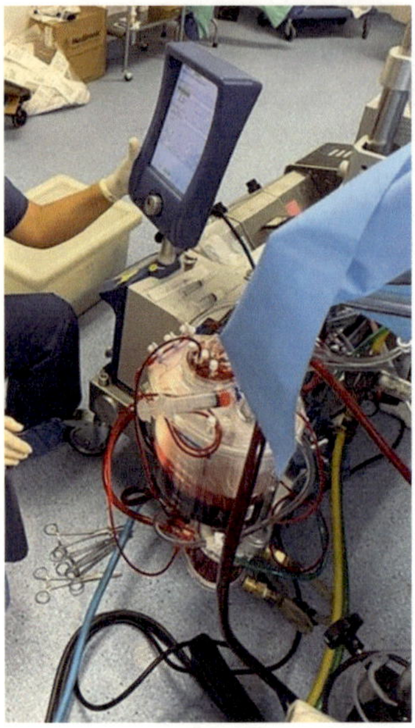

Figure 3.
Cardiopulmonary bypass (CPB).

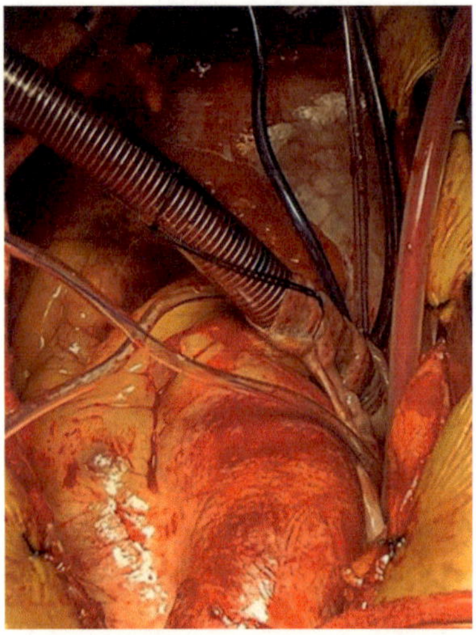

Figure 4.
Cannulation for CPB.

leukocyte-mediated factor generation, thus further increasing the local inflammatory response [26]. Likewise, if vasoactive substances are administered during surgery, they trigger the release of platelets that also respond to ECC or protamine administration, which can lead to pulmonary hypertension and systemic hypotension [27–29].

Also, secondary to complement activation, there is an increase in vascular permeability that may predispose the patient to capillary leak syndrome with fluid sequestration in the third space, particularly in the lung.

From a clinical perspective, the generalised inflammatory response results in postoperative pulmonary dysfunction, renal dysfunction and a resetting of the hypothalamic thermoregulatory centre [26, 28, 29–31].

This inflammatory response also has direct negative cardiac effects, as the inflammation caused by CPB involves platelet-endothelial cell interactions and vasospasm leading to low flow states in the coronary circulation. Anaphylatoxin C5a is a potent spasmogenic molecule and has leukocyte-activating properties that cause degranulation and release of oxygen free radicals [32]. Leukocytes exposed to complement are attracted to adhere to vascular endothelium and aggregate, resulting in vessel margination and leukoembolisation. These inflammatory cells mediate injury by increasing their production and releasing oxygen free radicals or proteolytic enzymes, a vicious circle, increasing the inflammatory state [33].

It is this release of oxygen free radicals that is generally implicated as the cause of transient postoperative ventricular dysfunction, which manifests approximately 2 hours after cessation of CPB and worsens 4–5 hours after CPB.

Recovery of ventricular function begins within 8–10 hours and full recovery usually occurs within 24–48 hours [34].

It is now known that systemic vascular resistance (SVR) increases as ventricular function worsens. This is a compensatory mechanism to maintain systemic blood pressure and perfusion in the face of depressed ventricular contractility. Oxygen free radicals and proteolytic enzymes released by neutrophils also damage endothelial cells, which increases capillary permeability and causes capillary leakage during this period and this increase in permeability lasts 2–3 days after surgery and is proportional to the duration of CPB [35].

On the other hand, uncontrolled hypothermia is also known to cause various alterations mainly in circulatory status, predisposing to cardiac arrhythmias, increasing SVR, precipitating shivering and altering coagulation. It indirectly decreases cardiac output by increasing vasoconstriction and causing bradycardia.

The CPB circuit is not the only factor responsible for this altered physiological state. Ischaemia and reperfusion time, hypothermia, hypotension with non-pulsatile flow, impaired coagulation and administration of blood and blood products are other factors contributing to the altered postoperative physiological state [36].

But there are important points in which all participants are involved, which are as follows:

3.7 Reduction of surgical site infections

It has always been a challenge for surgeons to minimise or abolish surgical site infections. Therefore different protocols have been developed including: topical intranasal therapy to eradicate *Staphylococcus aureus* colonisation; depilation protocols (an important measure in the cardiac patient), preferably cutting rather than shaving, which should be performed as close as possible to the time of surgery; proper management and timing of prophylactic antibiotic administration: 1st or 2nd generation cephalosporins (Level IA) are suggested to be administered no later than 1 hour before skin incision and should be continued up to 48 hours after surgery. If surgery lasts longer than 4 hours, additional doses should be administered in the operating room.

These manoeuvres have better results if combined with other previously mentioned manoeuvres such as smoking cessation, adequate glycaemic control and promotion of postoperative normothermia during recovery [16, 37].

3.8 Avoid hyperthermia

ECC can be performed under normothermic or hypothermic conditions. The efficiency of heat exchangers means that the patient may be subjected to inadvertent hyperthermia, especially during rewarming of a hypothermic CPB. Excessive hyperthermia during rewarming is defined as a core temperature > 37.9°C and is associated with increased postoperative neurological injury, infection and renal dysfunction [38].

3.9 Rigid sternal fixation

Most cardiovascular surgeons use wire cerclage to close the sternotomy, as it has a low rate of sternal wound complications and because of the low cost of the wires. Wire cerclage joins the cut edges of the bone by wrapping a wire or band around or through them and joining the two parts together. This achieves approximation and compression, but does not eliminate side-to-side movement and therefore rigid fixation is not 100% achieved.

More recently, sternal fixation with a rigid plate has been performed, which apparently provides significantly better sternal healing, with fewer sternal complications and no additional cost compared to wire cerclage at 6 months after surgery. Improvements include significant pain reduction, improved upper extremity function and improved quality of life, with no difference in overall cost.

Also, although these studies are still limited, the findings reported a lower rate of mediastinitis, decreased painful sternal pseudarthrosis after median sternotomy and superior bone healing compared to wire cerclage [39].

However, this remains a surgeon's decision but should be considered in special or high-risk patients, such as patients with a high body mass index, history of chest wall radiation, severe chronic obstructive pulmonary disorder or chronic steroid use.

Rigid sternal fixation may be useful to improve or accelerate sternal healing and reduce mediastinal complications [40, 41].

3.10 Management of bleeding and use of antifibrinolytics

Trans-surgical bleeding is one of the most common complications, as is bleeding greater than usual post-surgery. The range of reoperation varies from 0.69 to 7.8% and mortality increases by 15% if reoperation is performed [42, 43].

The administration of aminocaproic acid or tranexamic acid reduces the occurrence of major haemorrhage, as well as the need for less transfusion of blood products and the possibility of greater than usual bleeding or postoperative cardiac tamponade [44].

Currently, tranexamic acid is the most widely used, but it is associated with the presence of seizures, so it is recommended not to exceed a dose of 100 mg/kg body weight [45–47].

3.11 Surgical and/or haemodynamic decisions

During surgery, the big difference for an adequate recovery is the decision made for the exit of the CPB and its removal. In this area, the surgeon must decide, with the support of the anaesthesiologist, on different procedures, such as balloon counter pulsation in left ventricular failure, administration of vasoactive and/or inotropic agents or sometimes extracorporeal membrane oxygenation (ECMO).

4. Postoperative period

This period takes place in the intensive care unit (ICU), where protocols are already established (**Figure 5**).

Every patient admitted to the ICU has clinical problems that can change rapidly and the patient after open heart surgery is no exception [48, 49]. In fact, they are even more unpredictable. On admission, these patients are unstable and their clinical status is extremely fluid and dynamic. Care of the postoperative open heart patient requires the presence of healthcare staff at the bedside and must have knowledge of fundamental concepts of general care of the critically ill patient, as well as concepts specific to this group of patients. Initial management can set the tone for the remainder of the recovery period. Clinical errors at this time can have far-reaching implications.

Initial management should begin even before the patient arrives in the ICU. It is vital to know the medical history, previous indications for surgery, pre-operative haemodynamic data, comorbid conditions, medications and allergies [50].

Initial post-operative care in cardiac surgery requires a thorough physical examination and at least basic haemodynamic monitoring which should include: heart rate and rhythm, blood pressure, temperature, right and left heart filling pressures, haemodynamic profile, pharmacological and ventilatory support, chest drainage, assessment of neurological status, laboratory results, electrocardiogram and chest X-ray. A thorough knowledge of the specific monitoring and drug administration routes is essential, as well as having information on where the drains were placed. Once the initial assessment is complete, specific problems can be identified, prioritised and addressed [50, 51].

Subsequently, homeostasis of the internal environment should be restored, normothermia achieved, proper functioning of the epicardial pacemaker ensured and antibiotic prophylaxis continued.

It is essential to establish a multimodal analgesic strategy combining different analgesic families. This will help to reduce opioid doses, which will facilitate extubation, rehabilitation and early mobilisation of the patient.

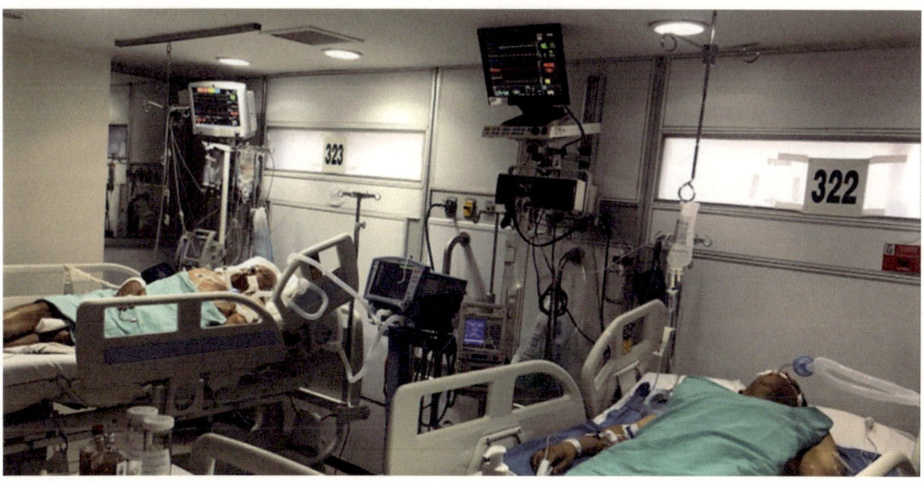

Figure 5.
Post-surgical intensive therapy unit.

Withdrawal of mechanical ventilation should be initiated when adequate haemodynamic stability is achieved. As in most patients, water resuscitation and actions to avoid probable acute renal failure should be administered; early initiation of thromboprophylaxis (mechanical and, when possible, pharmacological) and measures for the prevention of delirium should be given [50].

Resuscitation and haemodynamic management should be guided by objective parameters and advanced monitoring is indicated in those patients in whom there is instability, in whom it is necessary to investigate the pathophysiology of the evolution or in those patients who, due to their baseline characteristics, intraoperative evolution or the type of intervention, are considered a high surgical risk [52].

Advanced haemodynamic monitoring systems provide continuous information on more specific parameters, such as cardiac output and its determinants: preload or preload-dependence, contractility and afterload (**Figure 6**).

A total of 90% of all post-operative cardiac surgery patients present with transient low cardiac output (CO) related to the release of oxygen free radicals in response to the inflammatory state induced by CPB, (as explained above) or ischaemia/reperfusion injury due to cardioplegic arrest.

Low cardiac output (post-thoracotomy low cardiac output syndrome) is more common in women and when there is prolonged ECC time.

The aetiology of this syndrome may be preload, afterload, contractility or abnormal heart rate and rhythm or a combination of these.

The most common causes are related to decreased left ventricular preload caused by hypovolaemia and haemorrhage, vasodilatation, overheating, drugs, cardiac tamponade, right ventricular dysfunction, positive pressure ventilation and tension pneumothorax [50].

Increased afterload is usually the result of acute vasoconstriction, often related to vasoactive drug therapy. It may also be due to pre-existing hypertension, pain or sensitisation, fluid overload or hypothermia [50].

Decreased contractility is the main cause of low output in patients with pre-existing LV dysfunction associated with perioperative ischaemia. Perioperative ischaemia is often the consequence of poor intraoperative myocardial protection, incomplete revascularisation, coronary artery or coronary conduit spasm, coronary artery "junk"

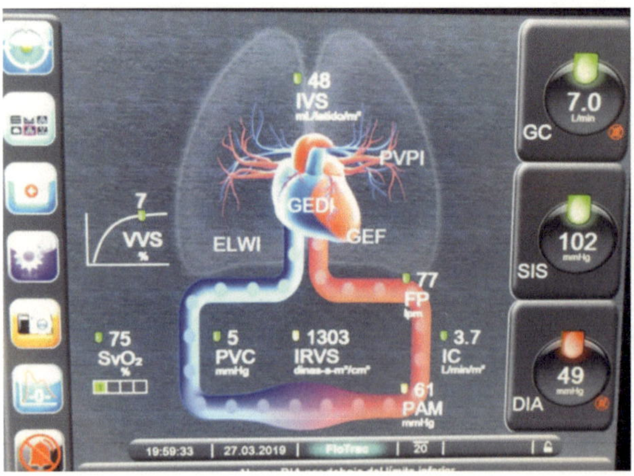

Figure 6.
Continuous haemodynamic monitoring in the ICU.

syndrome, graft closure (from any cause), acute anaemia (mainly bleeding) or the presence of hypoxia or acidosis of any aetiology [50].

Tachyarrhythmias negatively affect cardiac output by decreasing cardiac filling time and, consequently, coronary perfusion time of systolic volume. They also increase myocardial oxygen demand.

Bradyarrhythmias depress cardiac output, especially when left ventricular dysfunction limits the compensatory mechanism of increased stroke volume. Bradyarrhythmias are especially harmful in association with aortic insufficiency of any degree.

Atrial fibrillation results in loss of atrial contribution to cardiac output and a consequent fall in cardiac output.

Finally, any ventricular arrhythmia adversely affects cardiac output [50].

Contractility decreases in the immediate postoperative period of cardiac surgery compared to the preoperative period. The magnitude and duration of this phase depend on previous cardiac dysfunction, the existence of ischaemic events, preoperative complications and intraoperative evolution.

The elements that most affect cardiac dysfunction in this period are increased left ventricular mass or left ventricular dilatation, hypothermia, volume, route of cardioplegia administration and prolonged CPB time [53].

Two haemodynamic patterns may occur in the postoperative period that should be distinguished: (a) pressure overload (left hypertrophy and lusitropic dysfunction) which interferes with the assessment of filling pressures and may lead to an underestimation of volume requirements due to tachycardia intolerance; and (b) volume overload (typical in valvular regurgitation) which also alters the assessment of preload dependence and where the dynamic variables of volume response have not been validated.

Volume overload (typical in valvular regurgitation) which also alters the assessment of preload dependence and where dynamic volume response variables have not been validated.

Therefore, continuous assessment of volume response and its impact on haemodynamic parameters should be maintained to avoid inappropriate resuscitation [7].

To maintain adequate haemodynamic monitoring, there are different manoeuvres, from the placement of a flotation catheter and measurement of cardiac output and its variables to the performance of a transesophageal echocardiogram, which can be performed intraoperatively.

All these options are available in the ICU, including capillary filling, which is a validated, fast, reliable and safe technique to assess tissue perfusion in critically ill patients. As an integrator of multiple biological signals, it is a sensitive early warning system for a potentially lethal threat, activating according to the sum and intensity of the signals and turning off in the same direction.

Echocardiography has become a first-line tool in the evaluation of the postoperative patients with suspected major bleeding. As mentioned, it can be a transthoracic or transesophageal examination. Transthoracic echocardiography is of limited value in the immediate postoperative period due to the presence of wounds and their coverings and chest tubes, but it can provide some information on LV function and recognise obvious tamponade [54].

Transesophageal echocardiography is an extremely valuable tool as it provides excellent visualisation of cardiac dynamics, the pericardial space and the mediastinum. It is the best diagnostic modality for LV function, the presence of tamponade and the development of new valve abnormalities. It is also useful for the evaluation of the right ventricle [54].

Once the patient has been admitted to the unit and according to the patient's assessment and monitoring, the relevant vasoactive substances, inotropies and, conversely, vasodilators or antihypertensives will be initiated or continued as necessary.

However, all of the above strategies should be coupled with the following strategies, which have been studied and are related to the patient's improvement or deterioration in the postoperative period, whether or not they are implemented:

4.1 Perioperative glycaemic control

It is already well known that hyperglycaemia increases morbidity, which is multifactorial and attributed to glucose toxicity, increased oxidative stress, prothrombotic effects and pro-inflammatory effects. However, interventions to improve glycemic control are also known to improve in-hospital outcomes [55].

Preoperative carbohydrate loading has been shown to coincide with low glucose levels after a surgical procedure.

Epidural analgesia during cardiac surgery has also been shown to decrease the incidence of hyperglycaemia [56–58].

Treatment of hyperglycaemia (glucose >160–180 mg/dL) should preferably be done with post-cardiac surgery insulin infusion.

Postoperative hypoglycaemia should be avoided, especially in patients with an adjusted target blood glucose range (i.e., 80–110 mg/dL) [56–58].

4.2 Pain management

In the past, parenteral opioids were the mainstay of postoperative pain management. However, they are associated with multiple adverse effects, such as sedation, respiratory depression, nausea, vomiting and vertigo. It has now been shown that adequate pain management can be achieved through the additive or synergistic effects of different types of analgesics, allowing opioid doses to be reduced [59, 60].

NSAIDs are associated with renal dysfunction after cardiac surgery and selective COX-2 inhibition is associated with a significant risk of thromboembolic events.

The safest non-opioid analgesic is acetaminophen. When added to opioids, it has been found to produce superior analgesia, an opioid-sparing effect and independent antiemetic actions. The dose of acetaminophen is 1 g every 8 hours [61].

On the other hand, tramadol has opioid and non-opioid effects and, although it may be associated with a high risk of delirium, it decreases morphine consumption by 25%, resulting in adequate pain relief and increased postoperative patient comfort [62].

Pregabalin also reduces opioid consumption and is used in postoperative multimodal analgesia [63].

Dexmedetomidine, an intravenous α-2 agonist, reduces opioid requirements. Dexmedetomidine infusion has been shown to reduce 30-day cause-independent mortality, decrease the incidence of postoperative delirium and is associated with shorter intubation times [64].

4.3 Screening for postoperative delirium

Delirium is an acute confusional state characterised by mental status fluctuations, inattention and disorganised thinking or altered level of consciousness that occurs in approximately 50% of patients after cardiac surgery. It is associated with poorer in-hospital and long-term survival, hospital readmission and slower or reduced cognitive and functional recovery [9]. The cause is multifactorial, so early detection of delirium is critical to determine the underlying cause (pain, hypoxaemia, low cardiac output and/or sepsis) and initiate appropriate treatment [65].

Risk factors are many and include advanced age, recent alcoholism, preoperative organic brain syndrome, severe cardiac disease, multiple associated medical illnesses and prolonged time on CPB.

Common causes of delirium are drug toxicity, metabolic disorders, alcohol withdrawal, low cardiac output syndromes, periods of marginal cerebral blood flow during CPB, hypoxia, sepsis and recent stroke [9, 10].

Evaluation of delirium begins with a review of the patient's medications and inotropic/vasoactive levels, identification of the history of recent alcoholism or substance abuse, neurological examination and determinations of arterial blood gases, electrolytes, BUN, creatinine, blood biometry, magnesium and calcium.

Treatment of delirium begins with correction of any metabolic abnormalities, discontinuation of inappropriate medication and administration of psychotropic drugs for agitation, such as haloperidol, 2.5–5 mg OV/IV every 6 hours. Treatment of suspected alcohol withdrawal includes benzodiazepines, thiamine and folate.

Due to the complexity of the pathogenesis of delirium, more than one intervention must be performed, or more than one pharmacological agent may be necessary to diminish or control it. These medications include dexmedetomidine and olanzapine. Non-pharmacological strategies are a first-line component of treatment [66, 67].

4.4 Persistent hypothermia

Postoperative hypothermia is the inability to regain or maintain normothermia (36°C or greater) for 2–5 hours after admission to the ICU following cardiac surgery. Hypothermia is associated with higher than usual bleeding, infections, prolonged hospital stay and death. Prevention of hypothermia is necessary by using forced air warming blankets, increasing the ambient room temperature and avoiding the administration of cold solutions [68, 69].

4.5 Patency of mediastinal and/or pleural catheters

All patients undergoing cardiac surgery have mediastinal and/or pleural drains placed, as the thoracic cavity must be evacuated after surgery, as most patients have some degree of bleeding [70]. However, drains used to evacuate blood from the mediastinum tend to become clogged with clotted blood in up to 36% of patients and if this happens can cause tamponade or haemothorax.

However, retained mediastinal blood haemolyses promote an oxidative inflammatory process that can cause pleural and pericardial effusions and trigger postoperative atrial fibrillation [71].

Strategies for chest tube manipulation are varied and depend on the healthcare personnel performing the manipulation. However, any strategy should fragment visible clots and/or create short periods of high negative pressure to remove clots [72, 73].

On the other hand, higher than usual bleeding may be recorded precisely because of blood drainage by the same probes, which should be quantified on an hourly basis and, according to international guidelines, acted upon, either with transfusion (plasma, cryoprecipitates) or pharmacological measures (tranexamic acid, aminocaproic acid) or surgical re-intervention.

4.6 Thromboprophylaxis

Vascular thrombotic events include both deep vein thrombosis and pulmonary embolism and represent potentially preventable diseases.

All patients benefit from mechanical thromboprophylaxis achieved with compression stockings and/or intermittent pneumatic compression during hospitalisation or until they have adequate mobility to reduce the incidence of deep vein thrombosis after surgery even in the absence of pharmacological treatment [9, 73].

After cardiac surgery, these mechanical measures should be put in place, and prophylactic pharmacological anticoagulation should be initiated in 12–24 hours. After ICU admission, as satisfactory haemostasis must first be achieved, mainly at the thoracic level, and remember that CPB produces an inflammatory response that includes the coagulation system. Once adequate haemostasis is confirmed, pharmacological prophylaxis is initiated (most commonly on postoperative day 1 until patient discharge) [73, 74].

4.7 Extubation strategies

It is recommended to try to perform extubating early, preferably within 6 hours of the patient's arrival in the ICU. Protocols for extubating together with low-dose opioids are now available to enable such a procedure to be performed. This is safe (even in high-risk patients) and is associated with reduced ICU stay, reduced infections (pneumonia) and lower costs [9, 10, 75].

4.8 Acute kidney injury

Acute kidney injury (AKI) occurs in 22–36% of cardiac surgical procedures. Patients should be assessed on admission to identify those at risk of developing AKI, however, also the surgical procedure itself, the duration of CPB and hypotension/hypertensive events within the operating room can lead to AKI [76, 77]. Impaired renal oxygenation during CPB has been shown to improve with increased CPB flow but this may contribute to postoperative renal dysfunction and suggests the need to consider targeted perfusion strategies. It is therefore necessary to avoid nephrotoxic agents, to suspend angiotensin-converting enzyme inhibitors and angiotensin II antagonists for 48 hours, to maintain adequate blood volume and to avoid fluid overload and vasoplegic events. To avoid or prevent AKI, it is necessary to have strict control of creatinine and urine output, avoid hyperglycaemia and radiocontrast agents, as well as strict control to optimise hydration status and general haemodynamic parameters [78, 79].

When AKIN II-III acute kidney injury occurs, it is necessary to initiate renal replacement therapy, which is often with continuous slow haemodialysis (**Figure** 7).

4.9 Fluidotherapy

This manoeuvre uses monitoring techniques to guide the administration of fluids, vasopressors and inotropes to avoid hypotension and/or low cardiac output. This manoeuvre has quantified targets including blood pressure, cardiac index, mixed venous oxygen saturation and diuresis. In addition, oxygen consumption, oxygen debt and lactate levels can augment or modify therapeutic tactics.

Adequate volemia must be maintained without overload and must not be so low as to cause AKI [80].

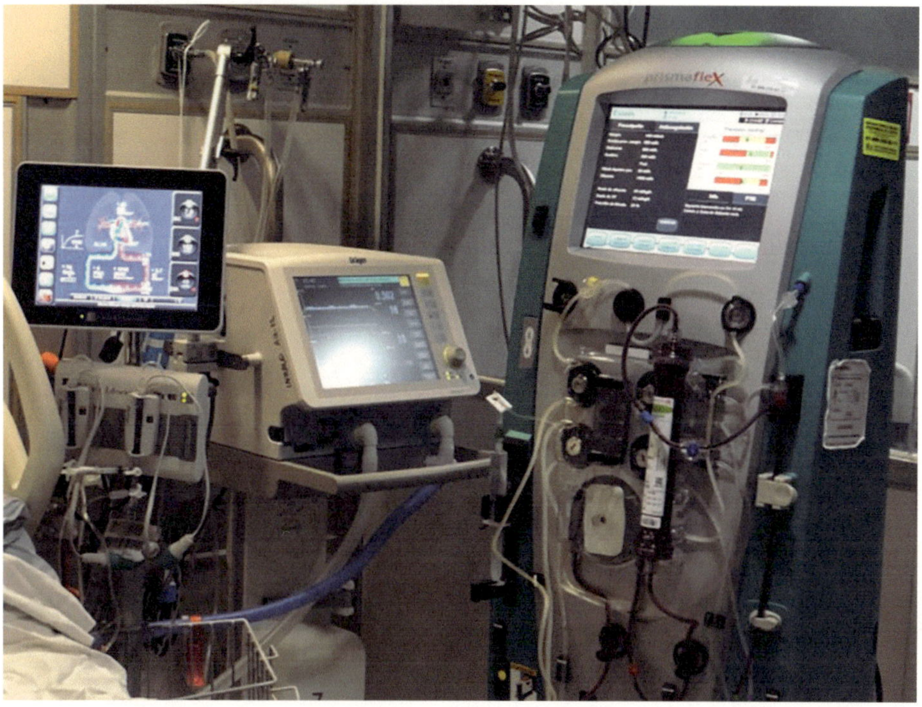

Figure 7.
Continuous slow dialysis therapy in the ICU.

4.10 Other factors

There is always the possibility of anaemia in the patient following cardiac surgery. The anaesthesiologist as well as the perfusionist perform manoeuvres to avoid severe anaemia, including transfusion of red blood cell concentrates, placement of cell salvage and/or haemofiltration during CPB. However, it is recommended to maintain a minimum haemoglobin level of 10 gm/dl in mainly ischaemic patients.

During mechanical ventilation, it is preferable to manage low tidal volume, as well as to maintain positive end-expiratory pressure (PEEP) at physiological levels and maintain measures for lung protection.

Early enteral nutrition should be considered, if haemodynamics and patient conditions allow.

Early mobilisation of the patient is also recommended, according to the patient's physical condition and possibilities [9, 19, 38].

There are also certain manoeuvres or devices that are placed in the operating room or within the ICU to maintain a better postoperative state or to improve shock, the presence of low post-thoracotomy output or immediate complications in surgical patients. This mechanical support is performed after pharmacological management either with vasoactive substances (noradrenaline, vasopressin) and/or inotropics (dobutamine, milrinone, levosimendan, etc.).

Intra-aortic balloon counterpulsation (IABP) is an effective tool for the treatment of low cardiac output states, ongoing ischaemia, valvular disease and the complications of myocardial infarction (**Figure 8**) [81].

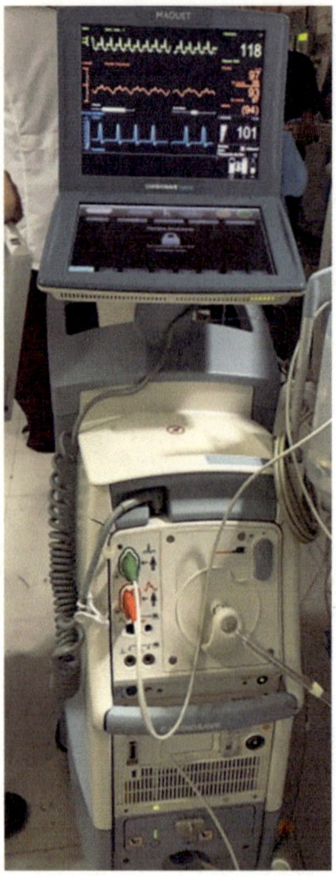

Figure 8.
Intra-aortic balloon pump.

This mechanism provides haemodynamic support and ischaemia control before and after surgery. It has been shown to be effective in improving left ventricular diastolic function. IABP is highly effective in the treatment of low cardiac output states. Unlike most inotropic agents, it provides haemodynamic support to the heart when myocardial oxygen demand is decreased and improves coronary artery perfusion, stabilising the myocardial oxygen supply: demand ratio [50].

It reduces the ejection impedance of the left ventricle by rapidly deflating just before systole, thereby unloading the LV and thus decreasing myocardial oxygen demand. As it rapidly inflates just after aortic valve closure, it increases diastolic coronary perfusion and improves myocardial oxygen delivery [50].

Indications for IABP placement are perioperative ischaemia, mechanical complications of myocardial infarction (such as acute mitral regurgitation, ventricular septal defect and cardiogenic shock), presence of greater than 80% left main coronary artery lesion in the preoperative period, postoperative low cardiac output states unresponsive to moderate doses of inotropics and acute deterioration of myocardial function to provide temporary support or a bridge to transplantation. IABP is contraindicated in the presence of aortic insufficiency, aortic dissection and severe aortic and peripheral vascular disease [50].

There are also circulatory or ventricular assist devices (VADs), which can be divided into right or left ventricular assist, however, these devices are not common in patients admitted after cardiac surgery [82]. They are the definitive therapy for low cardiac output. They are usually used intraoperatively when cardiopulmonary bypass disconnection is unsuccessful but may also be a postoperative option if the patient does not respond to vasoactive agents and IABP (**Figures 9** and **10**).

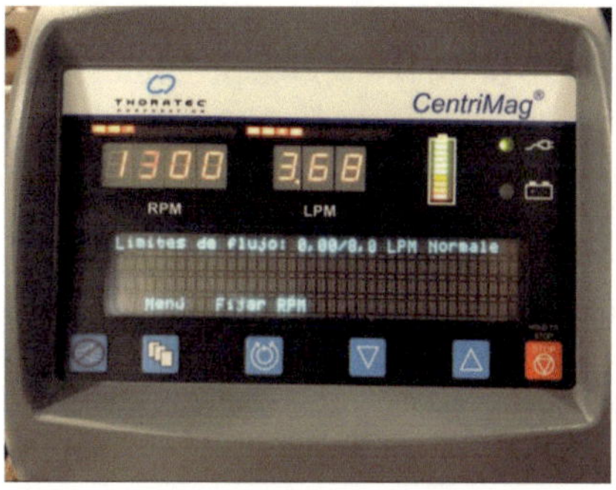

Figure 9.
Thoratec.

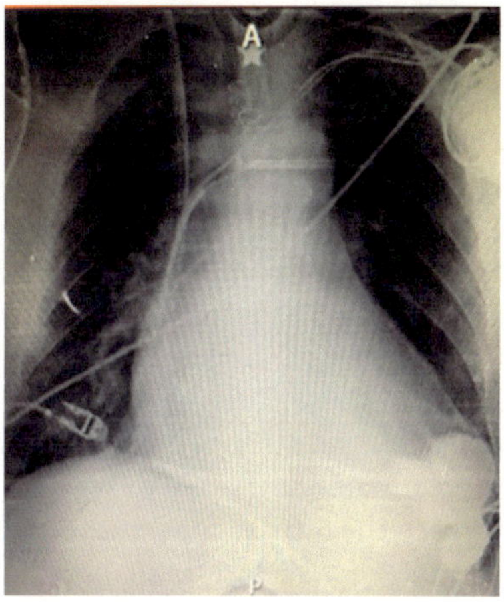

Figure 10.
Chest X-ray showing placement of heart mate III.

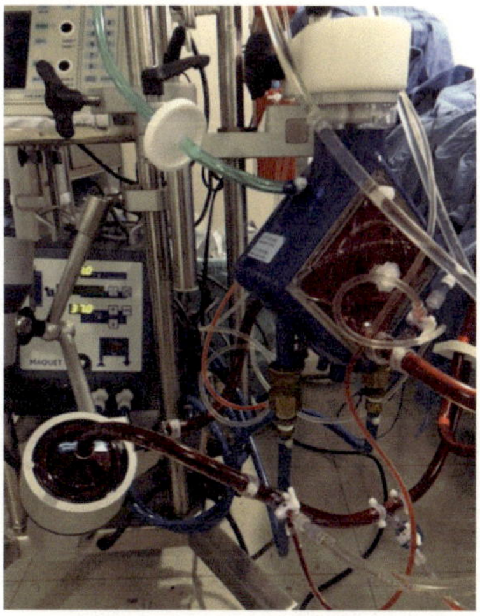

Figure 11.
ECMO.

General indications for VAD implantation include a complete and adequate cardiac surgical procedure, correction of all metabolic problems, inability to disconnect from cardiopulmonary bypass, inability to reverse haemodynamic deterioration despite maximal pharmacological therapy and IABP and a cardiac index less than 1.8–2 L/min/m^2 [82, 83].

To be optimally effective, circulatory assist devices to support low output require adequate lung function and gas exchange. In circumstances of compromised cardiac and pulmonary function, support of cardiopulmonary function is also required. Cardiopulmonary support (CPS) is achieved with a portable centrifugal pump, membrane oxygenator, heat exchanger and heparin-coated tubing. This system is generally referred to as extracorporeal membrane oxygenation (ECMO) (**Figure 11**). The indications for ECMO or SCP are the same as those for VADs in association with impaired oxygenation [50, 84, 85].

5. Conclusions

Cardiovascular surgery involves multiple manoeuvres and includes virtually all systems of the human body. Optimal perioperative management of interventional patients requires a comprehensive, multidisciplinary approach that includes adequate medical-surgical training. Preoperative optimisation, minimally invasive techniques, arrhythmia and postoperative bleeding prophylaxis, goal-directed haemodynamic management and multimodal analgesia allowing early extubation and mobilisation are key elements in the recovery of these patients.

The high level of complexity for the management, treatment and recovery of these patients makes intrinsic care units the ideal place to achieve the best results.

Close communication between the intensivist and the surgeon must be maintained to reduce the possibility of complications, treat them in a timely manner and ensure that the patient has an adequate evolution and subsequently improve their quality of life.

Author details

Maria del Carmen Renteria Arellano* and Hugo de Jesus Ballesteros Loyo
Angeles Lindavista Hospital, Mexico City, Mexico

*Address all correspondence to: mionyrent@gmail.com

References

[1] Ljungqvist O, Scott M, Fearon KC. Enhanced recovery after surgery: A review. JAMA Surgery. 2017;**152**(3):292-298. DOI: 10.1001/jamasurg.2016.4952

[2] Eskicioglu C, Forbes SS, Aarts MA, Okrainec A, McLeod RS. Enhanced recovery after surgery (ERAS) programs for patients having colorectal surgery: A meta analysis of randomized trials. Journal of Gastrointestinal Surgery. 2009;**13**(12):2321-2329. DOI: 10.1007/s11605-009-0927-2

[3] Lassen K, Soop M, Nygren J, et al. Consensus review of optimal perioperative care in colorectal surgery: Enhanced recovery after surgery (ERAS) group recommendations. Archives of Surgery. 2009;**144**(10):961-969. DOI: 10.1001/archsurg.2009.170

[4] Spanjersberg WR, Reurings J, Keus F, van Laarhoven CJ. Fast track surgery versus conventional recovery strategies for colorectal surgery. Cochrane Database of Systematic Reviews. 2011;**2**:CD007635

[5] Stone AB, Grant MC, Pio Roda C, et al. Implementation costs of an enhanced recovery after surgery program in the United States: A financial model and sensitivity analysis based on experiences at a quaternary academic medical center. Journal of the American College of Surgeons. 2016;**222**(3):219-225. DOI: 10.1016/j.jamcollsurg.2015.11.021

[6] Thiele RH, Rea KM, Turrentine FE, et al. Standardization of care: Impact of an enhanced recovery protocol on length of stay, complications, and direct costs after colorectal surgery. Journal of the American College of Surgeons. 2015;**220**(4):430-443. DOI: 10.1016/j.jamcollsurg.2014.12.042

[7] Jiménez Riveraa JJ, Llanos Jorgeb C, Gudec MJL, Velad JLP. Manejo perioperatorio en cirugía cardiovascular. Medicina Intensiva. 2021;**45**:175-183. DOI: 10.1016/j.medin.2020.10.006

[8] Grupo de trabajo de la Guía de Práctica Clínica sobre Cuidados Perioperatorios en Cirugía Mayor Abdominal. Guía de Práctica Clínica sobre Cuidados Perioperatorios en Cirugía Mayor Abdominal. Aragón, Spain: Ministerio de Sanidad, Servicios Sociales e Igualdad, Instituto Aragonés de Ciencias de la Salud (IACS); 2016. Guías de Práctica Clínica en el SNS

[9] Engelman DT, Ben Ali W, Williams JB, et al. Guidelines for perioperative care in cardiac surgery enhanced recovery after surgery society recommendations. JAMA Surgery. 2019;**154**(8):755-766

[10] Pokhrel SMD, Gregory AMD, Mellor AMD. Perioperative care in cardiac surgery. BJA Education. 2021;**21**(10):396-e402

[11] Schonborn JL, Anderson H. Perioperative medicine: A changing model of care. British Journal of Anaesthesia. 2019;**19**:27e33

[12] Snowden CP, Prentis J, Jacques B, et al. Cardiorespiratory fitness predicts mortality and hospital length of stay after major elective surgery in older people. Annals of Surgery. 2013;**257**:999-e1004

[13] Waite I, Deshpande R, Baghai M, et al. Home-based preoperative rehabilitation (prehab) to improve physical function and reduce hospital length of stay for frail patients undergoing coronary artery bypass graft and valve surgery. Journal of Cardiothoracic Surgery. 2017;**12**:91

[14] Tønnesen H, Nielsen PR, Lauritzen JB, Møller AM. Smoking and alcohol intervention before surgery: Evidence for best practice. British Journal of Anaesthesia. 2009;**102**:297e306

[15] Brady M, Kinn S, Stuart P. Preoperative fasting for adults to prevent perioperative complications. Cochrane Database of Systematic Reviews. 2003;**4**:CD004423

[16] Bustamante-Munguira J, Herrera-Gomez F, Ruiz-Alvarez M, Hernandez-Aceituno A, Figuerola-Tejerina A. A new surgical site infection risk score: Infection risk index in cardiac surgery. Journal of Clinical Medicine. 2019;**8**:480

[17] Edwards FH, Engelman RM, Houck P, Shahian DM, Bridges CR, Society of Thoracic Surgeons. The Society of Thoracic Surgeons practice guideline series: Antibiotic prophylaxis in cardiac surgery: Part I. Duration. The Annals of Thoracic Surgery. 2006;**81**:397-e404

[18] Wong J, Zoungas S, Wright C, Teede H. Evidence-based guidelines for perioperative management of diabetes in cardiac and vascular surgery. World Journal of Surgery. 2010;**34**(3):500-513. DOI: 10.1007/s00268-009-0380-0

[19] Kudsk KA, Tolley EA, DeWitt RC, et al. Preoperative albumin and surgical site identify surgical risk for major postoperative complications. JPEN Journal of Parenteral and Enteral Nutrition. 2003;**27**(1):1-9. DOI: 10.1177/014860710302700101

[20] Lee EH, Kim WJ, Kim JY, et al. Effect of exogenous albumin on the incidence of postoperative acute kidney injury in patients undergoing off-pump coronary artery bypass surgery with a preoperative albumin level of less than 4.0 g/dl. Anesthesiology. 2016;**124**(5):1001-1011. DOI: 10.1097/ALN.0000000000001051

[21] Karas PL, Goh SL, Dhital K. Is low serum albumin associated with postoperative complications in patients undergoing cardiac surgery? Interactive Cardiovascular and Thoracic Surgery. 2015;**21**(6):777-786

[22] Cameron D. Initiation of white cell activation during cardiopulmonary bypass: Cytokines and receptors. Journal of Cardiovascular Pharmacology. 1996;**27**(Suppl. 1):S1

[23] Tulla H, Takala J, Alhava E, et al. Hypermetabolism after cardiopulmonary bypass. The Journal of Thoracic and Cardiovascular Surgery. 1991;**101**:598

[24] Chiara O, Giomarelli PP, Biagioli B, et al. Hypermetabolic response after hypothermic cardiopulmonary bypass. Critical Care Medicine. 1987;**15**:995

[25] Crock PA, Ley CJ, Martin IK, et al. Hormonal and metabolic changes during hypothermic coronary artery bypass surgery in diabetic and non-diabetic subjects. Diabetic Medicine. 1988;**5**:47

[26] Chenoweth DE, Cooper SW, Hugli TE, et al. Complement activation during cardiopulmonary bypass: Evidence for generation of C3a and C5a anaphylatoxins. The New England Journal of Medicine. 1981;**304**:497

[27] Moore FD, Warner KG, Assousa S, et al. The effects of complement activation during cardiopulmonary bypass. Attenuation by hypothermia, heparin, and hem dilution. Annals of Surgery. 1988;**208**:95

[28] Dinarello CA. Interleukin-1 and the pathogenesis of the acute phase response. The New England Journal of Medicine. 1984;**311**:1413

[29] McCord JM, Wong K, Stokes SH, et al. Superoxide and inflammation: A mechanism for the anti-inflammatory activity of superoxide dismutase. Acta Physiologica Scandinavica. Supplementum. 1980;**492**:25

[30] Jastrzebski J, Sykes MK, Woods DG. Cardiorespiratory effects of protamine after cardiopulmonary bypass in man. Thorax. 1974;**29**:534

[31] Klausner JM, Morel N, Paterson IS, et al. The rapid induction by interleukin-2 of pulmonary microvascular permeability. Annals of Surgery. 1989;**209**:119

[32] Gold JP, Roberts AJ, Hoover EL, et al. Effects of prolonged aortic cross clamping with potassium cardioplegia on myocardial contractility in man. Surgical Forum. 1979;**30**:252

[33] Sladen RV, Berkowitz DE. In: Gravlee GP, Gavis RF, Uhey DR, editors. Cardiopulmonary Bypass and the Lung. 1st ed. Baltimore, MD: Williams & Willkins; 1993

[34] Przyklenk K, Kloner RA. "Reperfusion injury" by oxygen derived free radicals? Circulation Research. 1989;**64**:86

[35] Spiess BD. Ischemia-a coagulation problem? Journal of Cardiovascular Pharmacology. 1996;**27**(Suppl. 1):538

[36] Breisblatt WM, Stein KI, Wolfe CJ, et al. Acute myocardial dysfunction and recovery: A common occurrence after coronary bypass surgery. Journal of the American College of Cardiology. 1990;**15**:1261

[37] Edwards FH, Engelman RM, Houck P, Shahian DM, Bridges CR, Society of Thoracic Surgeons. The Society of Thoracic Surgeons practice guideline series: Antibiotic prophylaxis in cardiac surgery: Part I. Duration. The Annals of Thoracic Surgery. 2006;**81**:397-e404

[38] Engelman R, Baker RA, Likosky DS, et al. The society of thoracic surgeons, the society of cardiovascular anesthesiologists, and the American society of extra corporeal technology: Clinical practice guidelines for cardiopulmonary bypass temperature management during cardiopulmonary bypass. The Annals of Thoracic Surgery. 2015;**100**:748-e57

[39] Allen KB, Thourani VH, Naka Y, et al. Randomized, multicenter trial comparing sternotomy closure with rigid plate fixation to wire cerclage. The Journal of Thoracic and Cardiovascular Surgery. 2017;**153**(4):888-896.e1. DOI: 10.1016/j.jtcvs.2016.10.093

[40] Nazerali RS, Hinchcliff K, Wong MS. Rigid fixation for the prevention and treatment of sternal complications. Annals of Plastic Surgery. 2014; **72**(suppl. 1):S27-S30. DOI: 10.1097/SAP.0000000000000155

[41] Raman J, Lehmann S, Zehr K, et al. Sternal closure with rigid plate fixation versus wire closure: A randomized controlled multicenter trial. The Annals of Thoracic Surgery. 2012;**94**(6):1854-1861. DOI: 10.1016/j.athoracsur.2012.07.085

[42] Dyke C, Aronson S, Dietrich W, et al. Universal definition of perioperative bleeding in adult cardiac surgery. The Journal of Thoracic and Cardiovascular Surgery. 2014;**147**(5):1458-1463.e1. DOI: 10.1016/j.jtcvs.2013.10.070

[43] Ferraris VA, Brown JR, Despotis GJ, et al. 2011 update to the Society of Thoracic Surgeons and the Society of Cardiovascular Anesthesiologists blood

conservation clinical practice guidelines. The Annals of Thoracic Surgery. 2011;**91**(3):944-982. DOI: 10.1016/j.athoracsur.2010.11.078

[44] Myles PS, Smith JA, Forbes A, et al. ATACAS investigators of the ANZCA clinical trials network. Tranexamic acid in patients undergoing coronary-artery surgery. The New England Journal of Medicine. 2017;**376**(2):136-148. DOI: 10.1056/NEJMoa1606424

[45] Koster A, Faraoni D, Levy JH. Antifibrinolytic therapy for cardiac surgery: An update. Anesthesiology. 2015;**123**(1):214-221. DOI: 10.1097/ALN.0000000000000068

[46] Levy JH, Koster A, Quinones QJ, Milling TJ, Key NS. Antifibrinolytic therapy and perioperative considerations. Anesthesiology. 2018;**128**(3):657-670. DOI: 10.1097/ALN.0000000000001997

[47] Carl M, Alms A, Braun J, Dongas A, Erb J, Goetz A, et al. S3-Leitlinie zur intensivmedizinischen Versorgung herzchirurgischer Patienten: Hämodynamisches Monitoring und Herz-Kreislauf-System. GMS German Medical Science [Internet]. 2010;**8**:1-25. Disponible en: http://www.egms.de/static/de/journals/gms/2010-8/000101.shtml

[48] Pérez Vela JL, Martín Benítez JC, Carrasco González M, et al. Grupo de Trabajo de Cuidados Intensivos Cardiológicos y RCP de SEMICYUC. Clinical practice guide for the management of low cardiac output syndrome in the postoperative period of heart surgery. Medicina Intensiva. 2012;**36**:e1-e44. DOI: 10.1016/j.medin.2012.02.007

[49] O'Donnell JM, Nácul FE, editors. Posoperative care of the cardiac surgical patient. In: Surgical Intensive Care Medicine. 2010. pp. 535-566. DOI: 10.1007/978-0-387-77893-8_47

[50] Ochagavía A, Baigorri F, Mesquida J, et al. Hemodynamic monitoring in the critically patient. Recomendations of the cardiological intensive care and CPR working Group of the Spanish Society of intensive care and coronary units. Medicina Intensiva. 2014;**38**:154-169. DOI: 10.1016/j.medin.2013.10.006

[51] Habicher M, Zajonz T, Heringlake M, et al. S3-Leitlinie zur intensivmedizinischen Versorgung herzchirurgischer Patienten. Zeitschrift für Herz- Thoraxund Gefäßchirurgie [Internet]. 2018;**33**:40-44. Disponible en: http://link.springer.com/10.1007/s00398-018-0242-x

[52] Jiménez Rivera JJ, Llanos Jorge C, Iribarren Sarrías JL, Brouard Martín M, Lacalzada Almeida J, Pérez Vela JL, et al. Infused cardioplegia index: A new tool to improve myocardial protection. A cohort study. Medicina Intensiva. 2019;**43**:337-345. DOI: 10.1016/j.medin.2018.03.011

[53] Geisen M, Spray D, Nicholas FS. Echocardiography-based hemodynamic management in the cardiac surgical intensive care unit. Journal of Cardiothoracic and Vascular Anesthesia. 2014;**28**:733-744. DOI: 10.1053/j.jvca.2013.08.006

[54] Moghissi ES, Korytkowski MT, DiNardo M, et al. American association of clinical endocrinologists and American diabetes association consensus statement on inpatient glycemic control. Diabetes Care. 2009;**32**:1119e31

[55] Lazar HL, Chipkin SR, Fitzgerald CA, Bao Y, Cabral H, Apstein CS. Tight glycemic control in diabetic coronary artery bypass graft patients improves perioperative outcomes and decreases recurrent ischemic

events. Circulation. 2004;**109**(12):1497-1502. DOI: 10.1161/01.CIR.0000121747.71054.79

[56] Chaney MA, Nikolov MP, Blakeman BP, Bakhos M. Attempting to maintain normoglycemia during cardiopulmonary bypass with insulin may initiate postoperative hypoglycemia. Anesthesia and Analgesia. 1999;**89**(5):1091-1095. DOI: 10.1213/00000539-199911000-00004

[57] Gandhi GY, Nuttall GA, Abel MD, et al. Intensive intraoperative insulin therapy versus conventional glucose management during cardiac surgery: A randomized trial. Annals of Internal Medicine. 2007;**146**(4):233-243. DOI: 10.7326/0003-4819-146-4-200702200-00002

[58] White PF, Kehlet H, Neal JM, Schricker T, Carr DB, Carli F, et al. The role of the anesthesiologist in fast-track surgery: From multimodal analgesia to perioperative medical care. Anesthesia and Analgesia. 2007;**104**(6):1380-1396. DOI: 10.1213/01.ane.0000263034.96885.e1

[59] Wick EC, Grant MC, Wu CL. Postoperative multimodal analgesia pain management with nonopioid analgesics and techniques: A review. JAMA Surgery. 2017;**152**(7):691-697. DOI: 10.1001/jamasurg.2017.0898

[60] Jelacic S, Bollag L, Bowdle A, Rivat C, Cain KC, Richebe P. Intravenous acetaminophen as an adjunct analgesic in cardiac surgery reduces opioid consumption but not opioid-related adverse effects: A randomized controlled trial. Journal of Cardiothoracic and Vascular Anesthesia. 2016;**30**(4):997-1004. DOI: 10.1053/j.jvca.2016.02.010

[61] Radbruch L, Glaeske G, Grond S, et al. Topical review on the abuse and misuse potential of tramadol and tilidine in Germany. Substance Abuse. 2013;**34**(3):313-320. DOI: 10.1080/08897077.2012.735216

[62] Joshi SS, Jagadeesh AM. Efficacy of perioperative pregabalin in acute and chronic post-operative pain after off-pump coronary artery bypass surgery: A randomized, double-blind placebo controlled trial. Annals of Cardiac Anaesthesia. 2013;**16**(3):180-185. DOI: 10.4103/0971-9784.114239

[63] Ji F, Li Z, Young N, Moore P, Liu H. Perioperative dexmedetomidine improves mortality in patients undergoing coronary artery bypass surgery. Journal of Cardiothoracic and Vascular Anesthesia. 2014;**28**(2):267-273. DOI: 10.1053/j.jvca.2013.06.022

[64] Maldonado JR. Neuropathogenesis of delirium: Review of current etiologic theories and common pathways. The American Journal of Geriatric Psychiatry. 2013;**21**(12):1190-1222. DOI: 10.1016/j.jagp.2013.09.0

[65] Young J, Murthy L, Westby M, Akunne A, O'Mahony R, Guideline Development Group. Diagnosis, prevention, and management of delirium: Summary of NICE guidance. BMJ. 2010;**341**:c3704. DOI: 10.1136/bmj.c3704

[66] Page VJ, Ely EW, Gates S, et al. Effect of intravenous haloperidol on the duration of delirium and coma in critically ill patients (Hope-ICU): A randomised, double-blind, placebo-controlled trial. The Lancet Respiratory Medicine. 2013;**1**(7):515-523. DOI: 10.1016/S2213-2600(13)70166-8

[67] Karalapillai D, Story D, Hart GK, et al. Postoperative hypothermia and patient outcomes after elective cardiac surgery. Anaesthesia. 2011;**66**:780-784

[68] Engelen S, Himpe D, Borms S, et al. An evaluation of underbody forced-air and resistive heating during hypothermic, on-pump cardiac surgery. Anaesthesia. 2011;**66**(2):104-110. DOI: 10.1111/j.1365-2044.2010.06609.x

[69] Christensen MC, Dziewior F, Kempel A, von Heymann C. Increased chest tube drainage is independently associated with adverse outcome after cardiac surgery. Journal of Cardiothoracic and Vascular Anesthesia. 2012;**26**(1):46-51. DOI: 10.1053/j.jvca.2011.09.021

[70] St-Onge S, Perrault LP, Demers P, et al. Pericardial blood as a trigger for postoperative atrial fibrillation after cardiac surgery. The Annals of Thoracic Surgery. 2018;**105**(1):321-328. DOI: 10.1016/j.athoracsur.2017.07.045

[71] Day TG, Perring RR, Gofton K. Is manipulation of mediastinal chest drains useful or harmful after cardiac surgery? Interactive Cardiovascular and Thoracic Surgery. 2008;7(5):888-890. DOI: 10.1510/icvts.2008.185413 147

[72] Halm MA. To strip or not to strip? Physiological effects of chest tube manipulation. American Journal of Critical Care. 2007;**16**(6):609-612

[73] Kakkos SK, Caprini JA, Geroulakos G, et al. Combined intermittent pneumatic leg compression and pharmacological prophylaxis for prevention of venous thromboembolism. Cochrane Database of Systematic Reviews. 2016;**9**:CD005258

[74] Sachdeva A, Dalton M, Lees T. Graduated compression stockings for prevention of deep vein thrombosis. Cochrane Database of Systematic Reviews. 2018;**11**:CD001484

[75] Camp SL, Stamou SC, Stiegel RM, et al. Can timing of tracheal extubation predict improved outcomes after cardiac surgery? HSR Proceedings in Intensive Care and Cardiovascular Anesthesia. 2009;**1**(2):39-47

[76] Kashani K, Al-Khafaji A, Ardiles T, et al. Discovery and validation of cell cycle arrest biomarkers in human acute kidney injury. Critical Care. 2013;**17**(1): R25. DOI: 10.1186/cc12503

[77] Mayer T, Bolliger D, Scholz M, et al. Urine biomarkers of tubular renal cell damage for the prediction of acute kidney injury after cardiac surgery: A pilot study. Journal of Cardiothoracic and Vascular Anesthesia. 2017;**31**(6):2072-2079. DOI: 10.1053/j.jvca.2017.04.024

[78] Vanmassenhove J, Kielstein J, Jorres A, Biesen WV. Management of patients at risk of acute kidney injury. Lancet. 2017;**389**(10084):2139-2151. DOI: 10.1016/S0140-6736(17)31329-6

[79] Thomson R, Meeran H, Valencia O, Al-Subaie N. Goal-directed therapy after cardiac surgery and the incidence of acute kidney injury. Journal of Critical Care. 2014;**29**(6):997-1000. DOI: 10.1016/j.jcrc.2014.06.011

[80] Osawa EA, Rhodes A, Landoni G, et al. Effect of perioperative goal-directed hemodynamic resuscitation therapy on outcomes following cardiac surgery: A randomized clinical trial and systematic review. Critical Care Medicine. 2016;**44**(4):724-733

[81] Kantrowicz A, Tjonneland S, Freed PS, et al. Experiencia clínica inicial con bombeo intraaórtico para shock cardiogénico. Journal of the American Medical Association. 1968;**203**:113. DOI: 10.1001/jama.1968.03140020041011

[82] Pennington DG, editor. Mechanical circulatory support. Seminars in Thoracic and Cardiovascular Surgery. 1994;**6**:129-194

[83] Argenziano M, Oz MC, Rose EA. The continuing evolution of mechanical ventricular support. Current Problems in Surgery. 1997;**34**:318

[84] Smedira NG, Moazami N, Golding CM, et al. Clinical experience with 202 adults receiving extracorporeal membrane oxygenation for cardiac failure: Survival at 5 years. The Journal of Thoracic and Cardiovascular Surgery. 2001;**122**:92

[85] Smedira NG, Blackstone EH. Postcardiotomy mechanical support: Risk factors and outcomes. The Annals of Thoracic Surgery. 2001;**72**:S60

Chapter 6

Applying Person-Centered Care Model in the Postoperative Period of Renal Transplant Recipients: A Comprehensive Nursing Approach

Dilar Costa, Joana Silva and Jéssica Oliveira

Abstract

This study delves into the vital role of education in caring for kidney transplant recipients, underscoring the imperative for personalized, patient-centered educational programs. The analysis of nursing care quality standards, concerning health promotion, complication prevention, and autonomy, highlights the critical relevance of education in post-transplant management. Educational strategies, including participatory models and interdisciplinary approaches in the teaching process, are discussed. The conclusion underscores the nurse's pivotal role in comprehensively understanding the patient and effectively promoting resocialization after transplantation.

Keywords: kidney transplantation, nursing care, health education, self-care, quality of life

1. Introduction

Renal transplantation is considered the treatment of choice for end-stage renal disease (ESRD) [1]. Acknowledging its significance in ESRD treatment and its impact on the lives of those undergoing this intervention, we pose the question of the nurse's pivotal role in this field. The first query that arises is as follows: to what extent does this transformative process initiated by renal transplantation, introducing subsequent metamorphoses, qualitative ruptures, or any other notable discontinuities in the lives of kidney recipients, pose challenges, opportunities, and/or difficulties for nurses caring for these individuals in this critical period? The second inquiry seems to warrant phrasing in the following manner: what is the nurse's role in the success of renal transplantation, considering the risks and complications that the surgery entails? Before outlining, in broad terms, the response to these two questions, we allow ourselves to make the following observation: in this reflection on the nurse's role and the resources at their disposal to adequately address it, we are always part of a team of healthcare professionals contributing their expertise to achieve the intended outcome, namely, the effective functioning of the renal graft. In this regard, and already beginning to address the first question posed, Murphy [2] draws attention to the complexity, challenges, and rewards of nursing care for this population. The author delves into various activities within the nurse's competence defined in the nursing process. Starting with the assessment of the transplant recipient, we refer to its impact on gathering essential data for constructing an individualized care plan. Indeed, from the implementation of the nursing process in the postoperative period, the nurse works in multiple directions through specific guidelines, identifying problems, formulating diagnoses, defining expected outcomes and associated interventions, and assessing health gains for the person under their care [3, 4].

So, to start with one end of the issue, the care process begins with the patient's admission to the transplant unit after receiving a phone call from the hospital informing them that a kidney is available for them. Through precise instructions, the nurse responsible for the patient provides them with an overview of the scenario that awaits them in this period preceding the surgery. This information is rich in specifics about preoperative routines, extending to various spheres that constitute preoperative care: physical and psychological care, with special attention to the emotional and sociocultural spheres. Assessment is a relevant component as it encompasses the clinical, psychological, social, cultural, and economic history of the individual. The collection of these elements allows the nurse to easily describe the profile of the person in front of them, namely, assess functional capacity, describe the morphology of the support network, understand social status, habits, and lifestyles, the affective component, and know the services they use (community, health system, formal, and informal). Studies show that the success of kidney transplantation is directly related to the individual's health status and support network. This detailed assessment provides the foundation for formulating personalized care plans, centered on the individual needs and peculiarities of each recipient.

Some essential elements of the preoperative period underlying patient safety involve establishing a patient safety culture, defined as the set of best practices shared by healthcare professionals to prevent risks or harm to the patient in the pre, intra, and postoperative periods. This involves the adoption of protocols.

The postoperative period requires the implementation of preventive measures, early identification of potential complications, and patient education promotion. All these points are particularly relevant when considering the crucial role that the understanding and adherence of the transplant recipient assume in the success of kidney transplantation beyond the surgical act itself. From these elements emerges the care for the emotional state in response to the fears and anxieties of the transplant recipient facing the unknown world that has now begun. This attentive look acts as an effective device that guarantees the person's safety and protection in the face of present insecurity.

During this critical time, the nurse helps the person prepare to return home with tranquility and safety, which means adopting a patient and family-focused model.

The focus on the postoperative period goes beyond the necessary physical care for hemodynamic stability and the physical recovery of the transplant recipient. The answer to the second question is reflected in the paradigm shift and the investment in a new person-centered care model. If we observe its composition, we find that it aggregates physical/biological and psychosocial aspects, giving us a holistic and integrative view. The answer we have just outlined manifests, on the one hand, the structural axis of healthcare, which we could formalize around the dichotomies of person/health professionals, continuity/discontinuity, as the person, from our point of view, is the center of healthcare. Presently, the care system insists on the primacy of the person; its action is aimed at the individual and implicitly or explicitly asserts its primacy.

2. Person-centered care model for renal transplant recipients

The extent and significance of the person-centered care model vary across sociocultural contexts. In Europe, there is an appreciation for the person-centered care model, transcending the traditional healthcare approach by placing the individual at the core of care. This care model is more than a methodology; it is a philosophy that recognizes the unique attributes, preferences, and aspirations of each healthcare consumer. In the context of renal transplantation, the complexity and uniqueness of each individual highlight that person-centered care emerges as a guiding principle capable of meeting their physical, psychological, social, and cultural needs [5, 6].

One underlying reason for this choice is that, while the surgical act is crucial for the success of the transplant, the nurse's work represents a significant framework in the recovery of the transplant recipient. Infection prevention interventions, complication management, and health education promotion, including training in the management of immunosuppressive medication, also ensure the success of the surgery. Preparing the transplant recipient with the necessary adjustments for adaptation to the new reality mobilizes the material and emotional resources needed to live with the new organ. It also ensures the functions of protection, support, and assistance in transitioning back to family, professional, and social life in a new setting.

Available information indicates significant advancements in surgical techniques and immunosuppressive therapy, with renal transplantation being by far the most commonly performed surgical procedure in clinical practice [7].

All organ transplants are regulated by law. In Portugal, Law No. 12/93 of April 22 establishes the conditions related to the harvesting of organs and tissues of human origin. Its application extends to all Portuguese citizens, stateless individuals, and foreigners residing in Portugal [8].

The transplant can come from a living or deceased donor, and in Portugal, all citizens are considered potential post-mortem donors unless they express a contrary wish and are registered in the National Non-Donor Registry (RENNDA) [9].

According to data from the Portuguese Institute of Blood and Transplantation, in 2022, 495 kidney transplants were performed in Portugal. Observation of the records shows an increase in the overall donation rate between 2021 and 2022 (451 versus 495), similarly occurring in the first half of 2023 when compared with the corresponding period (223 versus 285) [10–12].

It is commonly accepted by authors that renal transplantation is the treatment of choice for end-stage renal disease in terms of survival and quality of life [13–16].

The success of renal transplantation needs to be viewed through the perspectives of different actors with diverse knowledge, concentrating and reinforcing their efforts in caring for the renal transplant recipient. Success will depend on the ability of these professionals to prepare the transplant recipient for adaptation and harmonious integration into the new context for an active life with the new organ. Questions about success arise positively. For example, how can this specific group and their families cope with the situation? How do we maximize the success of the renal graft? With which actors? Through what practices?

With the implementation of person-centered care, the aim is to generalize healthcare practices that respect the values and preferences of patients and promote their autonomy. Providing information, communicating, and educating are three essential aspects of this process. It is intended, from this care model, that the starting point be the needs and problems felt by individuals, their involvement in the therapeutic process, and in partnership with different healthcare professionals, facilitate healthy adjustment, culminating in the success of renal transplantation.

All of this leads to the consideration of actors as fundamental agents in the process, but above all, to imperatives of participation, interdisciplinary participation, and participation with the patient and family, and it is in this context that nurses play a central role in promoting and adapting the transplant recipient, helping to alleviate uncertainty and strengthen self-efficacy [16].

The transition from the surgical process to the post-transplant phase is marked by the beginning of a complex and challenging journey fraught with uncertainty, fear, and change. The role of the nurse gains prominence in promoting recovery and ensuring a healthy transition to the new reality of the renal transplant recipient.

Each interaction, each care provided, is permeated by an understanding of the unique goals, preferences, and challenges of renal transplantation. Taking person-centered nursing care as a reference, let us explore how these specific nursing interventions contribute to the success of renal transplantation in preventing risks and complications associated with surgery.

2.1 The person-centered care model

2.1.1 Definition and principles of person-centered care

The person-centered care model (PCCM) places the individual at the forefront of their care process and focuses on three main aspects: safety, education, and communication [17]. The concept itself takes on different terms to express similar principles and activities, such as holistic care, personalized care, among others [18]. Here, we understand the concept from the perspective of a holistic approach that considers the person in various dimensions: biological, psychological, social, and cultural.

In the context of renal transplantation, beyond the physical component associated with the surgical act, the psychological, social, and cultural components play a significant role in the individual's recovery and transition to the new reality. It all begins with empowering the person, giving them an active role, making it important to consider an individual-centered care model. Informed decision-making and support in disease self-management can improve the quality of care and health outcomes [18]. It is essential to understand the role of nurses in promoting care centered on the needs of the individual, based on their biological, psychological, and sociocultural needs. What is their degree of intervention, not only in interventions defined by nurses but also in the type of interventions they consider most suitable for the individual?

According to the Health Foundation, collaboration between the patient and healthcare professionals involves exploring what matters to the person and identifying the best treatment, care, and support. Thus, involving the person leads to better outcomes than "individual" decisions made by healthcare professionals. The nurse's support as a help system cannot be overlooked. Numerous factors, each playing a specific role, influence the care chain developed during the care process [18].

After renal transplantation, individuals face various challenges: physical, emotional, and social, need to deal with an increasing number of aspects related to transplantation, such as medication regimen, lifestyle changes, complications, infections, and adjustment to a new reality [19].

In short, there is intense turbulence caused by the new conditions. New resources, skills, and competencies are required to cope with the situation. At this moment, there is a crucial awareness of the need to rebalance life, which can only be achieved in its entirety by involving all individuals directly involved: the transplant recipient, family, and healthcare professionals. Such a strategy will only be viable through a person-focused care approach, aiming for the individual to develop the knowledge, skills, and abilities to make informed decisions and manage their therapeutic regimen [15].

The immediate question is: In the post-surgery period, what nursing interventions have been developed to care for the renal transplant recipient?

The part of nursing that addresses these issues falls under the competencies of nurses specializing in nephrology. According to the Portuguese Order of Nurses, nurses specializing in medical-surgical nursing (EEEMC) in the area of chronic disease are qualified to care for individuals with end-stage renal disease (ESRD) undergoing renal transplantation. The regulation proposed by the College of the Specialty of Medical-Surgical Nursing, approved in 2018, defines the specific competency profile of EEEMC, in addition to the common competencies of the nurse specialist defined in regulation n° 429/2018. The specific competencies include:

1. Caring for individuals/families/caregivers experiencing chronic illness, applying the nursing process, and developing specialized interventions.

2. Maximizing the therapeutic environment in collaboration with individuals/families/caregivers experiencing chronic illness [20].

The first point emphasizes partnership, safety, and quality of care, involving the identification of the needs of the individual and the family experiencing, in this particular case, a complex surgical process.

The second important point involves the prevention of complications and, in a broader approach, understanding the complexity of the situation experienced. The evaluation of the impact of surgery on the quality of life and well-being of the transplant recipient and their family is an area of intervention for the specialist nurse.

The activities developed in the next phase of the process aim to prepare the renal transplant recipient for the transition. Therefore, support for the transplant recipient and their family is crucial for obtaining favorable health outcomes. The post-transplant period is challenging in that the individual moves toward a new path fraught with uncertainties and potential complications [21].

Cooperation between the transplant recipient, their family, and the nurse brings benefits when a commitment is made to undertake the best strategies for promoting, preventing, and managing the disease. It is hoped that the individual gains skills through learning experiences promoted by the nurse, develop abilities for managing the new condition, and can find solutions to detected problems. Thus, the appreciation of the potential of the individual and their family is positive and adds value to the therapeutic relationship.

In this regard, and to give an idea of the relevance of the specialist nurse in caring for the renal transplant recipient and their family, we highlight two key aspects of their responsibility: the safety of the patient and the quality of nursing care, which, although transversal to all nurses, have greater weight for the specialist nurse and are part of their competencies, as can be consulted in the regulation of specific competencies of the EEEMC in the area of chronic disease. This includes preventing complications and adverse events resulting from the disease, managing the therapeutic environment, promoting a safe and quality environment in the provision of nursing care, and preventing and controlling infections, both within the healthcare team and by assisting the patient and their family in adhering to infection prevention and control behaviors [22].

On the agenda, the issue that gains visibility in the field of renal transplantation is the quality of life of renal transplant recipients, involving the incorporation of knowledge about the disease (a circumstance that, according to some authors, may be at the root of a disturbing beginning due to the unfamiliarity of how to deal with the new situation) and how to manage it.

After transplantation, the individual remains hospitalized for an average of five to ten days before being discharged home [23]. During this hospitalization period, various events can occur, such as post-surgery complications, for example, deep vein thrombosis, paralytic ileus, bleeding, renal artery thrombosis, urinary fistula, lymphocele, infection, pain, and rejection, among others [24].

The rate of major complications after transplant surgery is low and has a very small contribution to graft loss, but it requires the attention of the nurse [25]. A rigorous assessment of the patient is essential to prevent and/or minimize complications. Thus, considering the need to ensure the safety of the individual, promote effective recovery, prevent complications, and facilitate the transition to an active life with the new organ, specific nursing interventions are needed. This leads us to the following question: what care do nurses promote in the postoperative period for the renal transplant recipient?

In the next section, we answer this question.

3. Applying person-centered care in the postoperative phase

3.1 Postoperative care nursing interventions

The context of nursing interventions during the postoperative and recovery period involves various essential actions. By explicitly focusing on the contribution of nurses in this scenario, we cannot overlook other critical elements, especially in the context of renal transplantation. A fundamental aspect is preparing the individual for the return home, aligning with the principles of the ontology of nursing care. In this context, there is an opportunity to develop a holistic approach that considers the individual as a whole, addressing physical, emotional, social, and spiritual aspects.

The integration of health education in this context emerges as the essential link to empower transplant recipients to live fully with the new organ. Focusing on preparing for the return home and adopting a holistic approach establishes the bridge of health education as a strategic element of a cognitive process aimed at empowering the individual for self-management of their condition, providing them with extensive knowledge about living with the renal graft. This allows the individual to be the subject of their own journey.

Health education, as a tool for teaching and learning, gives mastery to the patient and enables them to become autonomous subjects capable of making informed decisions. Indeed, a crucial aspect of education is aligned with the individual's individual needs, recognizing them as an active and capable entity. Thus, health education not only informs but also empowers, aligning with the holistic and person-centered vision that guides the entire care process in the field of transplantation.

The generated debate, markedly directed toward the recovery period and the preparation of the renal transplant individual for the return to normality, not only highlights their role as the main actor in this process but also emphasizes optimizing the success of transplantation through education, however, without intending to relegate the crucial relevance of the biological aspect in postoperative care.

According to the literature, the implementation of the Enhanced Recovery After Surgery (ERAS) protocol in the preoperative, intraoperative, and postoperative periods promotes patient recovery, reduces the risk of complications, facilitates early discharge, and reduces healthcare costs [26].

Studies indicate that the implementation of ERAS is well-established in various surgical areas but is a relatively new concept in renal transplantation [27–30]. However, its application in renal transplantation has shown benefits for the patient. In a study by Dias et al., the authors developed and implemented the standardized ERAS protocol in 200 transplanted patients, of which 100 were subjected to the protocol and the other 100 to standard care. The study took place between 2017 and 2018, and the outcomes of interest were the length of hospital stay, the incidence of delayed graft dysfunction, and the readmission rate. The results showed, in the experimental group, a shorter average length of hospital stay than the control group by 2 days (the average length of hospital stay in the experimental group was 5 days and in the control group was 7 days), and for 79% of participants in the experimental group, discharge occurred on the fourth postoperative day. The rate of delayed renal function was similar in both groups, as was the readmission rate. For the authors, the implementation of the ERAS protocol, in addition to being essential, is safe since there was no increase in the complication rate and/or delayed renal graft function [31].

Another study allowed us to verify the benefits of ERAS in renal transplantation. The authors included 286 renal transplant recipients, of which 135 underwent the recovery program, and 156 received standard care. The study's objective was the application of ERAS principles and measuring changes in quality of life and satisfaction with care. The results showed a lower use of morphine for postoperative pain management in the experimental group compared to the control group and statistically significant (median was 9.5 vs. 47 mg; $P > 0.001$). Similar to the previous study, the authors also obtained a shorter average length of hospital stay in the experimental group than in the control group (median was 5 days vs. 7 days; $P < .001$). Unlike the study by Dias et al., the authors found in the experimental group a readmission rate of less than 5% in the 10 days following transplantation [32].

If the above-described view of the benefits of the ERAS protocol in renal transplantation seems like a path to follow, based on research confirmed in the literature, this new approach, albeit recent in the field of renal transplantation, is highly stimulating if we think about the challenge of responding, through models and strategies, to the uncertainties, fears, concerns, and needs of renal transplant individuals.

The principles underlying this approach are those of a person-centered approach, so they can be easily adapted to renal transplantation. A multidisciplinary team consisting of surgeons, anesthesiologists, intensivists, nephrologists, nurses, and other healthcare areas involved in care for renal transplant individuals, such as a nutritionist, radiologist, pharmacist, social worker, etc., is involved in the entire process. The transplant recipient is involved in this process [33].

The program encompasses three stages: stage 1, the period preceding surgery; stage 2, the period immediately before surgery; stage 3, the immediate recovery period corresponding to the period of preparing the individual for discharge, that is, helping the individual leave the hospital as soon as possible if well prepared and ensuring support at home after hospital discharge [34].

This is an evidence-informed approach aimed at minimizing the stress caused by surgery and helping the individual recover quickly. However, its implementation remains challenging and should be adapted to each patient [35].

This framework, already theorized in various disciplinary fields, should be problematized in the context of renal transplantation as a reference framework for caring for renal transplant individuals.

The ERAS approach includes three domains, as mentioned earlier: preoperative, intraoperative, and postoperative. Since our focus is on the postoperative period, the recommended actions for this phase encompass many nursing interventions developed by the nurse during this period, such as:

- Rigorous monitoring, through constant monitoring of vital signs.
- Monitoring renal function with special attention to diuresis. Significant changes may indicate graft dysfunction or rejection. Monitoring laboratory values such as creatinine and urea.
- Pain control and multimodal analgesia.
- Early mobilization. Prevention of deep vein thrombosis and pulmonary embolism. This may also involve the administration of low molecular weight heparin, if prescribed by the medical team.
- Adequate hydration and nutrition. On the first day after surgery, initiate a liquid diet, progressively evolving to a solid diet according to tolerance.
- Control of nausea and vomiting.
- Complications. After a transplant, patients face a myriad of potential postoperative complications. These include surgical complications such as wound infections, bleeding, or organ damage, as well as the risk of viral, bacterial, and fungal infections due to the immunosuppressive medications required to prevent organ rejection. Additionally, there's a constant concern for graft dysfunction and organ rejection, which can manifest as a decline in organ function or outright rejection by the recipient's immune system. Moreover, patients may also encounter other complications such as neoplasms and cardiovascular issues, further emphasizing the importance of vigilant post-transplant care and monitoring.
- Infection prevention. Removal of medical devices (urinary catheter, drains) as soon as the clinical condition allows (on average, they remain for 5 to 7 days). Surveillance of the surgical site, implementation of infection prevention and control measures such as hand hygiene.
- Immunosuppression.
- Emotional support.
- Promotion of autonomy.
- Patient education [36].

This set of actions corresponds to the quality standards of nursing care (PQCE) defined by the Order of Nurses, namely health promotion, prevention of complications, well-being and self-care, and functional readjustment. A study conducted in Brazil analyzed postoperative care for kidney transplant recipients based on the perception of 10 nurses. According to the participants, the interventions in their clinical practice for this group include monitoring vital parameters, infection prevention with particular attention to hand hygiene, hydration, diuresis monitoring (Fluid Balance), immunosuppressive medication, pain control, and monitoring complications. Anxiety is also a central focus of their care. The discharge plan is not part of their routine [37].

However, the hospital discharge plan is a fundamental element in preparing the individual for home and is essential in promoting autonomy. Standardized discharge plans contribute to increasing self-care capacity, communication between the nurse and the patient, and preventing hospital readmission. Post-transplantation requires the individual to manage their disease concerning symptom management, medication, complications, and infections. This fact leads us to consider health education as a key factor in promoting self-care in disease management [38].

In reality, the need to respond quickly to the situation created by the transplant challenge highlights education as a fundamental component in preparing the individual for home. During hospitalization, the transplant recipient and their family learn how to care for their renal graft. Building on the PQCE defined by the Order of Nurses, the nurse helps the individual achieve the maximum health potential. Thus, in line with the goals set with the individual, particularly regarding self-care, the nurse creates and seizes opportunities to promote identified healthy lifestyles. Additionally, they provide information that promotes cognitive learning and the development of new capabilities by the individual [22].

The promotion of autonomy involves preparing the patient and their family, as mentioned earlier, and education is a valuable tool from the perspective of requirements for hospital discharge. A review study on nursing care in the postoperative period of renal transplantation highlights education as an important factor in the success of renal transplantation [39].

The relationship between self-care and health outcomes is close. The educational process directed at the transplant recipient and their family regarding self-care behaviors is essential for effective management of their health condition. It is due to this need that education is considered the cornerstone in caring for this specific group [24].

After transplantation, individuals need to learn to manage a complex medication regimen, monitor the side effects of therapy, monitor signs of rejection and infection, and deal with complications and comorbidities [40].

Investing in education is understood as a means to equip the individual with the essential tools for self-management. Support also plays a significant role in this learning process [41]. What education strategies can be developed in the transplant scenario to prepare for the return home?

In the next section, we address education as one of the pathways to transplant success.

4. Patient education for self-care

In the normal sequence of actions to ensure the success of surgery and the quality of life for transplant recipients, several authors have outlined education programs aimed at kidney transplantation. The choice of participatory education models takes into account the degree of importance attributed to individuals in managing their illness process. This scenario includes a randomized clinical trial conducted in 2018 in Tabriz, Iran, involving 60 hospitalized kidney transplant recipients at the Iman Reza Hospital. The authors implemented and evaluated the effectiveness of a self-care education program for this population.

The study aimed to develop and implement an education program based on the needs of this specific group to assist them in resolving emerging problems and improving their quality of life. Initially, researchers administered a questionnaire to participants to identify their needs. Subsequently, they developed the education program, consulting a nephrologist beforehand. Education sessions were conducted at the patient's bedside and lasted for 30 to 45 minutes. Three sessions were provided to the experimental group. Researchers used a book as a resource for the education session, covering concepts and definitions of the disease, medication, dietary regimen, physical exercise, and self-care activities. The results showed statistically significant differences between the two groups after administering the education program, particularly in self-care and quality of life. In the domain of self-care education, the experimental group had, on average, higher scores than the control group after the educational sessions (average scores in self-care and quality of life between the two groups: EG = 6.017 vs. CG = 5.175; $p > .001$). They concluded that the education program is effective in improving knowledge about kidney transplantation and quality of life. They emphasize the role of nurses in promoting the knowledge and skills necessary for disease management [42].

Several studies emphasize the nurse's role in preparing transplant recipients for their new condition. Training should be seen as a means of support for change, and in this perspective, nurses play a fundamental role [2, 13].

Some studies clearly demonstrate that education should be tailored to the individual's background to promote successful learning, with the teach-back model proving crucial for ensuring learning success [43–45].

Interdisciplinarity is fundamental in the educational process, contributing to the education of transplant recipients. Nowadays, it is challenging for transplant education to be confined to a single discipline due to various constraints related to knowledge development, technological advancement, and the individual needs of the person. The nurse's assumption of this role does not imply that other healthcare professionals are entirely excluded from this process. Nurses are with patients 24 hours a day, providing them with more time to understand their physical and psychological needs, including motivation and readiness to learn [2].

The involvement of the patient remains undeniably crucial, especially when they will be responsible for managing their health condition. Changes after transplantation will undoubtedly influence what is learned, how it is learned, and even the stereotypes constructed about the disease. Some studies suggest that many patients struggle with managing their illness because they are unaware of the relevance of their participation in the process and how to handle the complexity associated with the situation. One of the nurse's functions is to inform the person about the challenges and complications that the situation brings. Transplant recipients need to acquire knowledge about immunosuppressive medication, monitor signs of rejection, and understand the benefits of changing certain lifestyle styles [46].

Urstad and colleagues [47] demonstrate in their study the effect of an educational intervention on the knowledge, adherence, self-efficacy, and quality of life of kidney transplant recipients. They conducted a randomized clinical study involving 139 participants, with 77 in the experimental group and 82 in the control group. Various measurement instruments were applied (knowledge questionnaire, SF-12, self-efficacy scale, and observation). Measurements took place between the 7th and 8th weeks post-transplant.

Statistically significant differences were found between the two groups in terms of knowledge in both assessment periods ($p = 0.002$ and $p = 0.004$). Similarly, self-efficacy scores differed between the two groups in both assessments, with the experimental group showing higher values than the control group ($p = 0.036$), and the quality of life followed the same direction ($p = 0.001$). The authors concluded that a personalized education program tailored to the individual positively influences knowledge, self-efficacy, and quality of life.

This leads us to the following question: what to include in the education program? Based on the literature, we have defined some contents that we consider relevant for the teaching/learning process, namely:

1. Personalized and Individualized Education

    - Consider specific characteristics of the individual, such as health literacy levels, particularly regarding kidney transplantation, cultural preferences, and medical history.

2. Competency-Based Education

    - Focus on the competencies necessary for self-care, enabling the acquisition of skills/capabilities needed to manage their condition.

3. Incorporation of Technology

    - Incorporate innovative technologies, such as mobile applications or online platforms, to facilitate real-time access to information. They can serve as a means of continuous support and easy access to educational resources.

4. Involvement of the Family

    - Involving the family in the educational process, besides providing emotional support, plays an active role in helping the person adhere to recommendations.

5. Proactive Approach to Potential Complications

    - Include information on warning signs of possible post-transplant complications and teach proactive management of any abnormal symptoms that may arise.

6. Continuous Assessment of the Individual's Understanding

    - Continuous assessments should be conducted to identify any cognitive changes that may compromise the ability to learn and manage the disease.

In our view, education sessions should address immunosuppressive medication, self-care (monitoring renal function, urinary output, blood pressure, temperature, weight, and capillary blood glucose if clinically indicated, surveillance for signs of rejection and potential infections), healthy lifestyles, vaccination, and sexuality.

Another important aspect is the establishment of personalized goals, effective communication, follow-up, and continuous support.

The transition to kidney transplantation requires an adaptation period that necessitates communication, a teaching pace tailored to each individual's rhythm, the encouragement of a strong dynamic with spaces for dialog, a space to respect and integrate cultural differences, and also different personalities.

It is essential to give space for transplant recipients and their families to participate in the project, starting by listening to their priorities and expectations, trying to understand their logics, and then preparing them for any challenges that the disease may bring.

5. Conclusion

What can be concluded?

The nurse caring for kidney transplant recipients faces daily challenges that cannot be ignored. Therefore, for the success of kidney transplantation, it is important to develop a comprehensive understanding of transplantation and the lives of those being cared for: who they are, how they live, with whom they live, what their concerns, worries, beliefs, expectations, religion, and cultural context are. Knowing each of these facets in their interactions with the individual and their family helps to obtain a holistic view of the whole that characterizes them and develop personalized/individualized education programs.

Education is an important factor in teaching/learning and should follow a standardized, person-centered structure. In fact, individuals with chronic kidney disease need to reintegrate into society once transplanted, and most are on an equal footing in terms of knowledge and disease self-management skills. Success lies in adherence to the therapeutic regimen in its various aspects. Studies show that the better-adapted group is the one that learns to cope with the disease and experiences fewer difficulties.

In this context, the nurse's role is crucial to overcoming difficulties and providing transplant recipients with the necessary tools for a healthy adaptation. Education should be considered an essential and never secondary element because, as we have seen, it is through education that better openness to socializing with kidney transplantation is achieved, and the self-efficacy and autonomy of the transplant recipient are built.

Conflict of interest

The authors declare no conflict of interest.

Author details

Dilar Costa*, Joana Silva and Jéssica Oliveira
Unidade Local de Saúde Santa Maria, Lisbon, Portugal

*Address all correspondence to: dilarcosta@gmail.com

References

[1] Rocha CCT, da Neto AV, da Silva AB, Farias VA, Junior AD, da Silva RA. Cuidados de enfermagem ao paciente transplantado renal: scoping review. Aquichan. 2021;**21**(3):e2136-e2136. Available from: https://aquichan.unisabana.edu.co/index.php/aquichan/article/view/16019/6539

[2] Murphy F. The role of the nurse post-renal transplantation. The British Journal of Nursing. 2007;**16**(11):667-675. DOI: 10.12968/bjon.2007.16.11.23689

[3] Gaffuri T, Zanella KA, Marolli C, Silva. Renal transplantation: Intensive therapeutic nurse in the immediate post-operative. Revista de Pesquisa: Cuidado é Fundamental Online. Aug 2020;**20**:1144-1149

[4] Chapman JR. The recipient of a renal transplant. In: Hebert MJ, Prasad GV, Jutzeler CR, editors. Kidney Transplantation – Principles and Practice. Alemanha: Springer; 2019

[5] Magee CC, Pascual M. Update in renal transplantation. Archives of Internal Medicine. 2004;**164**(13):1373-1388. DOI: 10.1001/archinte.164.13.1373

[6] Barbosa MM, Afonso RM, Paúl C, Lezaun JY. Cuidados Centrados na Pessoa Idosa em Portugal: Abordagens e instrumentos de avaliação. In: Abstract presented at: Actas do 13° Congresso Nacional de Psicologia da Saúde; 2020 Jan-Feb 30-1; Covilhã.

[7] Kellar CA. Solid organ transplantation overview and delection criteria. The American Journal of Managed Care. 2015;**21**(Suppl. 1):S4-S11

[8] Portugal. Ministério Público. Lei n.° 12/93, de 22 de abril de 1993. Diário da República n.° 94/1993, Série I-A de 1993-04-22

[9] IPST, IP - RENNDA [Internet]. www.ipst.pt. Available from: https://www.ipst.pt/index.php/pt/rennda

[10] Instituto Português do Sangue e da Transplantação, IP. Dados Anuais Atividade de Doação e Transplantação 2021. Acedido a 10 de setembro 2023. Disponível em: https://www.ipst.pt/files/TRANSPLANTACAO/DOACAOETRANSPLANTACAO/Dados_Anuais_Atividade_Doacao_Transplantacao2021_versao_integral_para_publicacao.pdf

[11] Instituto Português do Sangue e da Transplantação, IP. Dados Anuais Atividade de Doação e Transplantação 2021. Acedido a 10 de setembro 2023. Disponível em: https://www.ipst.pt/files/TRANSPLANTACAO/DOACAOETRANSPLANTACAO/DadosAnuaisAtividadeDoaaoTransplantacao2022Apresentacaorevista.pdf

[12] Instituto Português do Sangue e da Transplantação, IP. Dados Anuais Atividade de Doação e Transplantação 2021. Acedido a 10 de setembro 2023. Disponível em: https://www.ipst.pt/files/TRANSPLANTACAO/DOACAOETRANSPLANTACAO/ AtividadeColheitaTransplantacaoOrgaos_1Sem__2023v2.pdf

[13] McPake D, Burnapp L. Caring for patients after kidney transplantation. Nursing Standard. 2009;**23**(19):49-57. DOI: 10.7748/ns2009.01.23.19.49.c6744

[14] Demet D, Aksoy N, Kiraz N. Nursing care after kidney transplant: Case report. Experiment in Clinical Transplantation.

2018;**16**(Suppl. 1):55-60. DOI: 10.6002/ect.TOND-TDTD2017.O22 Retraction in: Exp Clin Transplant. 2018 Jun;16(3):357. PMID: 29527993

[15] van Zanten R, van Dijk M, van Rosmalen J, Beck D, Zietse R, Van Hecke A, et al. Nurse-led self-management support after organ transplantation-protocol of a multicentre, stepped-wedge randomized controlled trial. Trials. 2022;**23**(1):14. DOI: 10.1186/s13063-021-05896-0

[16] The European Society for Organ Transplantation. Transplant nursing research in Europe. 2021. Available from: https://esot.org/wp-content/uploads/2021/04/Transplant-Nursing-Research-in-Europe-compressed.pdf

[17] Enes JE. A patient-Centered care model. Radiologic Technology. 2011;**82**(3):212. Available from: https://web.p.ebscohost.com/ehost/pdfviewer/pdfviewer?vid=51&sid=c8616b6e-4b42-48c0-8c9b-09ba82f811f0%40redis [Accessed: November 2022]

[18] The Health Foundation. Person-centred Care Made Simple [Internet]. The Health Foundation. Jan 2016. Available from: https://www.health.org.uk/sites/default/files/PersonCentredCareMadeSimple.pdf

[19] Serra A, Simões A, Fernandes J, Ferreira M. O Cuidado Centrado Na Pessoa Ebook Escola Superior De Saúde Egas Moniz Monte Da Caparica 2021 [Internet]. Available from: https://comum.rcaap.pt/bitstream/10400.26/37866/1/EBOOK%20II%20JEESSEM%202020.pdf

[20] Portugal. Ordem dos Enfermeiros. Regulamento de Competências Especificas do Enfermeiro Especialista em Enfermagem Médico-Cirúrgica: Na área de Enfermagem à Pessoa em Situação Crítica. 2017

[21] Lerret SM, Weiss ME, Stendahl G, Chapman S, Neighbors K, Amsden K, et al. Transition from hospital to home following pediatric solid organ transplant: qualitative findings of parent experience. Pediatric Transplantation. 2014;**18**(5):527-537. DOI: 10.1111/petr.12269

[22] Portugal. Ordem dos Enfermeiros. Regulamento n. ° 429/2018. Diário da República, 2.ª série, N. ° 135 de 16 de julho de 2018. 19359-19370. 2018

[23] Mahdizadeh A, Oskouie F, Khanjari S, Parvizy S. The need for renovating patient education in kidney transplantation: A qualitative study. Journal of Education Health Promotion. 2020;**30**(9):154. DOI: 10.4103/jehp.jehp_574_19

[24] Trevitt R, Dunsmore V, Murphy F, Piso L, Perriss C, Englebright B, et al. Pre- and post-transplant care: Nursing management of the renal transplant recipient: Part 2. Journal of Renal Care. 2012;**38**(2):107-114. DOI: 10.1111/j.1755-6686.2012.00302.x

[25] Jung GO, Chun JM, Park JB, Choi GS, Kwon CH, Joh JW, et al. Clinical significance of posttransplantation vesicoureteral reflux during short-term period after kidney transplantation. Transplantation Proceedings. 2008;**40**(7):2339-2341. DOI: 10.1016/j.transproceed.2008.06.027

[26] Jaszczuk S, Natarajan S, Papalois V. Anaesthetic approach to enhanced recovery after surgery for kidney transplantation: A narrative review. Journal of Clinical Medicine. 2022;**11**(12):3435. DOI: 10.3390/jcm11123435

[27] Halawa A, Rowe S, Roberts F, Nathan C, Hassan A, Kumar A, et al. A better journey for patients, a better

deal for the NHS: The successful implementation of an enhanced recovery program after renal transplant surgery. Experimental and Clinical Transplantation. 2018;**16**(2):127-132. DOI: 10.6002/ect.2016.0304

[28] Ricotta C, Cintorino D, Pagano D, Bonsignore P, Piazza S, di Francesco F, et al. Enhanced recovery after implementation of surgery protocol in living kidney donors: The ISMETT experience. Transplantation Proceedings. 2019;**51**(9):2910-2913. DOI: 10.1016/j.transproceed.2019.04.089

[29] Angelico R, Romano F, Riccetti C, Pellicciaro M, Toti L, Favi E, et al. The enhanced recovery after surgery (ERAS) pathway is a safe journey for kidney transplant recipients during the "extended criteria donor" era. Pathogens. 2022;**11**(10):1193. DOI: 10.3390/pathogens11101193

[30] Majumder A, Fayezizadeh M, Neupane R, Elliott HL, Novitsky YW. Benefits of Multimodal Enhanced Recovery Pathway in Patients Undergoing Open Ventral Hernia Repair. Journal of the American College of Surgeons. Jun 2016;**222**(6):1106-1115

[31] Dias BH, Rana AA, Olakkengil SA, Russell CH, Coates PTH, Clayton PA, et al. Development and implementation of an enhanced recovery after surgery protocol for renal transplantation. ANZ Journal of Surgery. 2019;**89**(10):1319-1323. DOI: 10.1111/ans.15461

[32] Elsabbagh AM, Ghoneim I, Moiz A, Welch K, Brown JS. Enhanced recovery after surgery pathway in kidney transplantation: The road less traveled. Transplantation Direct. 2022;**8**(7):e1333. DOI: 10.1097/TXD.0000000000001333

[33] Zhang X, Yang J, Chen X, Du L, Li K, Zhou Y. Enhanced recovery after surgery on multiple clinical outcomes: Umbrella review of systematic reviews and meta-analyses. Medicine (Baltimore). 2020;**99**(29):e20983. DOI: 10.1097/MD.0000000000020983

[34] Kruszyna T, Niekowal B, Kraśnicka M, Sadowski J. Enhanced recovery after kidney transplantation surgery. Transplantation Proceedings. 2016;**48**(5):1461-1465. DOI: 10.1016/j.transproceed.2015.11.037

[35] Altman AD, Helpman L, McGee J, Samouëlian V, Auclair MH, Brar H, et al. Society of Gynecologic Oncology of Canada's communities of practice in ERAS and venous thromboembolism. Enhanced recovery after surgery: Implementing a new standard of surgical care. CMAJ. 2019;**191**(17):E469-E475. DOI: 10.1503/cmaj.180635

[36] Golder HJ, Papalois V. Enhanced recovery after surgery: History, key advancements and developments in transplant surgery. Journal of Clinical Medicine. 2021;**10**(8):1634. DOI: 10.3390/jcm10081634

[37] Santana RS, Silva FJA, Santos JS, Batista CA, Frota CA, Morais MJ, et al. Nursing care to patients in postoperative renal transplant. Rev Pre Infec e Saúde. 2019;**5**:9064. Available from: http://www.ojs.ufpi.br/index.php/nupcis/article/view/9064. DOI: 10.26694/repis.v5i0.9064

[38] Suzuki VF, Carmona EV, Lima MH. Planejamento da alta hospitalar do paciente diabético: construção de uma proposta [Planning the hospital discharge of patients with diabetes: the construction of a proposal]. Rev Esc Enferm USP. 2011;**45**(2):527-532. DOI: 10.1590/s0080-62342011000200032

[39] Cunha TGS, Lemos KC. Assistência de enfermagem às fases do transplante

renal: uma revisão integrativa. Health Residencies Journal. 2020;**1**:8. DOI: 10.51723/hrj.v1i8.143

[40] Driscoll A, Davidson P, Clark R, Huang N, Aho Z. Tailoring consumer resources to enhance self-care in chronic heart failure. Australian Critical Care. 2009 Aug;**22**(3):133-140. DOI: 10.1016/j.aucc.2009.05.003

[41] Murphy F. Managing post-transplant patients in primary care. Practice Nursing. 2011;**22**(6):292-297

[42] Aghakhani N, Maslakpak MH, Jalali S, Parizad N. Self-care education program as a new pathway toward improving quality of life in kidney transplant patients: A single-blind, randomized, Controlled Trial. Experiment in Clinical Transplantation. 2021;**19**(3):224-230. DOI: 10.6002/ect.2020.0044

[43] Mollazadeh F, Hemmati Maslakpak M. The effect of teach-back training on self management in kidney transplant recipients: A Clinical Trial. International Journal of Community Based Nursing Midwifery. 2018;**6**(2):146-155

[44] Côté J, Fortin MC, Auger P, Rouleau G, Dubois S, Boudreau N, et al. Web-based tailored intervention to support optimal medication adherence among kidney transplant recipients: Pilot parallel-group randomized controlled trial. JMIR Form Research. 2018;**2**(2):e14. DOI: 10.2196/formative.9707

[45] Andersen MH, Wahl AK, Engebretsen E, Urstad KH. Implementing a tailored education programme: Renal transplant recipients' experiences. Journal of Renal Care. 2019 Jun;**45**(2):111-119. DOI: 10.1111/jorc.12273

[46] Ponticelli C, Graziani G. Education and counseling of renal transplant recipients. Journal of Nephrology. 2012;**25**(6):879-889. DOI: 10.5301/jn.5000227

[47] Urstad KH, Wahl AK, Andersen MH, Øyen O, Hagen KB. Limited evidence on the effectiveness of educational interventions for kidney transplant recipients. Results of a Systematic Review of Controlled Clinical Trials. Patient Education and Counseling. Feb 2013;**90**(2):147-154

Chapter 7

Neuropsychiatric Morbidities in Non-Cardiac Surgical Patients Related to Perioperative Anaesthesiologic and Intensive Care

Clemens Kietaibl

Abstract

This book chapter provides neuropsychiatric morbidities related to perioperative patient care including both surgeries under general or regional anaesthesia and postoperative intensive care. While detailed guidelines have been already developed for the perioperative care for patients with cardiac comorbidities, guidelines for patients with pre-existing neuropsychiatric morbidities are currently limited. In particular, these limitations may affect non-cardiac surgical and non-neurosurgical patients, which is why it seems important to develop treatment guidelines which are applicable to patients undergoing major general surgeries under general or regional anaesthesia including postoperative intensive care. Hence—although provided neuropsychiatric aspects and morbidities related to anaesthesiologic perioperative patient care are applicable to all surgical disciplines—the provided treatment recommendations primarily apply to patients undergoing general surgeries.

Keywords: neuropsychiatric morbidities, perioperative anaesthesiologic care, non-cardiac surgical patients, postoperative intensive care, perioperative treatment recommendations

1. Introduction

This book chapter initially describes important neuropsychiatric morbidities primarily in general surgical patients including delirium, postoperative cognitive dysfunction (POCD), postoperative posttraumatic stress disorder (PTSD), perioperative stroke, convulsive status epilepticus (CSE) and non-convulsive status epilepticus (NCSE), cerebral macro- and microangiopathy, Alzheimer's disease (AD), cerebral autoregulation dysfunction and limited cognitive reserve (CR). Subsequently, identifying perioperative patients with underlying neuropsychiatric morbidities is specified. Finally, treatment recommendations for perioperative anaesthesiologic care of non-cardiac surgical patients with neuropsychiatric morbidities are described including both surgeries under general or regional anaesthesia and postoperative intensive care.

2. Neuropsychiatric morbidities in patients undergoing non-cardiac surgeries

2.1 Potential difficulties in the perioperative care of non-cardiac surgical patients

While anaesthesiologists usually have based on evidence-based guidelines an explicit concept for patients with pre-existing cardiac morbidities, potentially limited guidelines for patients with pre-existing neuropsychiatric morbidities may complicate perioperative anaesthesiologic care [1]. Concerning neuropsychiatric morbidities, degenerative cerebral morbidities based on cerebral macro- and microangiopathy may play the most significant role due to their high prevalence in general surgical patients. These patients frequently have a reduced cerebral perfusion, a disturbed cerebral autoregulation and an impaired carbon dioxide (CO_2) reactivity [2].

In Europe around 19 million of patients undergo mid-sized or major surgeries—worldwide around 200 million of patients. Perioperative complication rates are about 7–11%, with a mortality rate of about 0.8–1.5%, whereby cardiac complications show the highest frequency (about 42%) [3]. While cardiac complications have been exactly investigated, the pathophysiology underlying neuropsychiatric complications is currently poorly explored—supposing a multifactorial pathophysiology including a potentially surgically induced systemic inflammatory response syndrome (SIRS) with subsequent neuroinflammation [4–6].

2.2 Postoperative delirium

The incidence of postoperative delirium varies within a wide range from 5 to 65% [5]. Since delirium significantly increases perioperative morbidity, mortality and the duration of hospital stay [7], it is important for anaesthesiologists to know specific risk factors for postoperative delirium. Firstly, predisposing risk factors include a high patient age, hypertension, alcohol- and nicotine abuse, sleep disturbances, vision and hearing disorders, sensory disturbance, pain, limited exposition to daylight, infections, physical immobilisation, social isolation, abstinence syndrome, dehydration, electrolyte and acid-base imbalance, metabolic disorders, seizures and critical illness requiring postoperative intensive care [8]. In addition, a pre-existing cerebral impairment—in particular, dementia—seems to be a major risk factor [7, 9]. Obviously, some of these pre-existing risk factors may be also applicable to intra- and postoperative patient care. Secondly, specific risk factors related to surgeries and perioperative anaesthesiologic care are polytrauma, emergency surgeries, medically induced coma, mechanical ventilation, high blood loss, blood transfusion, hypoxaemia and temperature fluctuations [6, 8]. Finally, considering postoperative intensive care, treatment with extracorporeal circulations—in particular venoarterial extracorporeal membrane oxygenation (ECMO)—may tend to increase the incidence of overall neuropsychiatric morbidities including postoperative delirium [10].

The cardinal symptoms of delirium are spatial and temporal disorientation and impaired attention. Since postoperative patients regularly may be hypoactive and lethargic—and these symptoms could be assigned to a preceding general anaesthesia, dementia or depression—especially a hypoactive delirium remains undetected at times [7]. In particular regarding postoperative intensive care, although clinical tests for delirium are currently increasing, a relatively high number of undetected postoperative delirium probably exist [6].

The assumed pathophysiology underlying postoperative delirium is primarily a cerebral neuroinflammation impairing the blood-brain barrier (BBB) based on a SIRS potentially induced by surgical stress. According to current knowledge, a multifactorial pathophysiology seems probable [6]. Concerning that up to 50% of patients with postoperative sepsis have delirium, microvascular alterations, metabolic disturbances and impaired aerobic processes probably contribute significantly to the multifactorial pathophysiology [11]. Moreover, significant intraoperative blood pressure fluctuations are associated with delirium, while the role of intraoperative hypotensive time periods remains a bit unclear [12]. Whereas specific medications used in the perioperative period (e.g. benzodiazepines, opiates, propofol, glucocorticoids and atropine) may promote delirium, dexmedetomidine seems being protective [8]. However, whether using regional anaesthesia instead of general anaesthesia to reduce delirium-associated medications decreases the occurrence of postoperative delirium remains currently unproven—one reason for this might be the complex pathophysiology [13]. The latest research investigates postoperative blood pressure regulation—suggesting that particularly postoperative hypotensive periods contribute to delirium and overall patient morbidity and mortality [14, 15].

2.3 Postoperative cognitive dysfunction (POCD)

POCD is characterised as a subtle decline in patient's cognitive ability from its preoperative baseline including the following specific cognitive domains: learning and memory, language, perceptual-motor, social cognition, complex attention and executive function. In contrast to immediate cognitive impairment potentially related to multiple causes (e.g. recovery from anaesthesia or surgery, pain, anxiety and sleep disturbance), POCD onset starts several days later and may last for months or even years. POCD can significantly affect the quality of life, potentially outweighing the surgical benefits, which has more serious sequelae in the elderly population. In addition, POCD is associated with a higher postoperative 1-year mortality [16]. Finally, in particular, the elderly population should be perioperatively examined by multiple psychometric tests for POCD [17].

POCD occurs most often after cardiac (up to 80%), orthopaedic (up to 60%) and major general surgeries (up to 50%) [16, 18]. Specifically, after non-cardiac surgeries, the occurrence of POCD in patients with advanced age lies after 1 week, about 30%, after 3 months, about 13% and after 1 year, about 1%. Primary risk factors for POCD include a high age, a low educational level, pre-existing cerebrovascular or cardiovascular diseases and cognitive dysfunction at hospital discharge. Further risk factors may be a pre-existing cerebral impairment, prolonged anaesthesia and surgery, revision surgeries, postoperative infections and respiratory complications [16, 17].

The pathophysiology underlying POCD is currently not completely understood—a cerebral neuroinflammation potentially due to surgical stress-inducing cholinergic dysfunction and neuronal death seems to play a key role [17]. In addition, the exposition to cerebral microemboli—gaseous or solid—may contribute to POCD [18]. Cerebral microemboli exposition may occur in non-cardiac surgical patients primarily during major orthopaedic surgeries [18] and postoperative intensive care, if patients are treated with extracorporeal circuits—in particular, venoarterial ECMO may generate a high load of cerebral microemboli (**Figure 1**) [10].

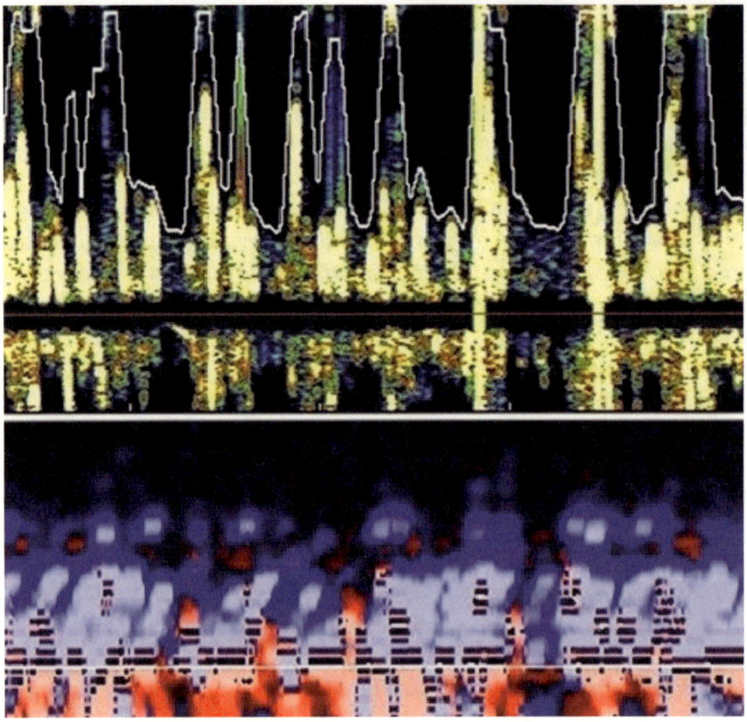

Figure 1.
Cerebral microemboli during venoarterial extracorporeal membrane oxygenation. The yellow spots represent a high load of cerebral microemboli in the middle cerebral artery using transcranial Doppler ultrasound.

Clinicians often believe that regional anaesthesia may reduce the incidence of POCD compared to general anaesthesia. However, current research could not prove a reduction of POCD using regional anaesthesia—in particular considering prolonged POCD [16]. While electroencephalography (EEG) guided total intravenous anaesthesia (TIVA) based on propofol seems being protective, clinical variables including hypoxia, hypotension and impaired cerebral perfusion could not be certainly associated with POCD [17]. Due to neuroprotective effects, dexmedetomidine is suggested to reduce POCD, whereas the potential benefits of ketamine and non-steroidal anti-inflammatory medications are currently unclear [8, 17]. Finally, keeping the postoperative hospital stay as short as possible consecutively returning the patient to everyday life may decrease a prolonged POCD [16].

2.4 Postoperative posttraumatic stress disorder (PTSD)

PTSD is generally characterised by behavioural avoidance, negative thoughts or mood and impaired physical or emotional reactions. Concerning young children (≤6 years), clinical symptoms may additionally include simulating the traumatic event during playing and frightening dreams commonly related to the traumatic event. In addition, symptoms may be aggravated by disturbed sleep patterns, frequent flashbacks, panic attacks and suicidal thoughts. The onset of postoperative PTSD may start within 1 month after surgery and may last for years—the intensity of symptoms typically varies related to peoples' baseline stress level or coming across the event.

The quality of life may be significantly impaired by social withdrawal, disability to carry out work or normal daily tasks and worse relationships [19–21].

In non-cardiac surgical patients, PTSD occurs frequently after major general surgeries (4–53%). The following perioperative risk factors for PTSD could be identified: intraoperative awareness (>2 minutes), postoperative intensive care, delirium, sepsis and SIRS [22, 23]. While most pre-existing neuropsychiatric morbidities increase the occurrence of postoperative PTSD, preoperative depression seems having protective effects [21]. Referring to benzodiazepines, intraoperative usage is protective due to their amnestic effects reducing intraoperative awareness [22], whereas benzodiazepines during postoperative intensive care may trigger PTSD [19]. According to current knowledge, a cerebral neuroinflammation potentially based on a SIRS may play a key role in the pathophysiology of PTSD [21].

The diagnosis of postoperative PTSD should consist of a physical examination and a psychiatric evaluation 2–6 hours, 2–36 hours and 30 days after surgery to identify also a prolonged onset of PTSD—using the criteria in the fifth edition of the Diagnostic and Statistical Manual of Mental Disorders (DSM-5) [24, 25]. Magnetic resonance imaging (MRI) research showed in PTSD patients reduced volumes of the hippocampus, the amygdala and the anterior cingulum [26].

The multifactorial treatment of PTSD currently prefers fast recovery concepts [27]. Most important is psychotherapy including cognitive and behavioural therapy. In addition, medical therapy consists of antidepressants (e.g. selective serotonin reuptake inhibitors, sertraline and paroxetine), anti-anxiety medications and prazosin in case of nightmares. A further application of anti-inflammatory drugs might be a promising option in the future. Moreover, treatment includes therapeutic exercise and nutritional therapy. Finally, eye movement desensitisation and reprocessing (EMDR) represent an additional modern therapy [27, 28].

2.5 Perioperative stroke

Perioperative stroke with clinical symptoms is a rare complication of general surgeries during the operation and postoperatively within 30 days (0.08–0.7%). However, since perioperative stroke is associated with a high mortality rate (18–26%) exceeding the mortality rate of strokes in the general population, it ranks among the most important neuropsychiatric perioperative complications [29, 30]. In contrast, perioperative silent strokes—strokes without any noticeable symptoms—have an incidence of up to 7% [31]. They typically affect a small part of the brain which is not necessary for vital functions. Hence, perioperative silent strokes regularly remain clinically undetected, but they can be diagnosed by MRI.

Risk factors for perioperative strokes in non-cardiac surgical patients are a high age, a pre-existing stroke or transient ischaemic attack (TIA), myocardial infarction within 6 months before surgery, atrial fibrillation, hypertension, hypercholesterolaemia, nicotine abuse, acute renal failure, dialysis and chronic obstructive pulmonary disease (COPD) [30].

Perioperative stroke is defined as brain infarction of ischaemic or haemorrhagic aetiology occurring during or within 30 days after surgery [32]. The majority is of ischaemic origin primarily based on either cardioembolisms - caused by atrial fibrillation or right-to-left shunt - or on embollisms due to vulnerable atherosclerosis of the aortic arch. Further ischaemic reasons include cerebral hypoperfusion, cerebral artery thrombosis and combined aetiologies. Although intraoperative hypotension may be less frequently associated with stroke than previously assumed, the perioperative ischaemic evaluation (POISE) trial showed a positive correlation between beta-blocker-induced intraoperative hypotension or bradycardia and perioperative stroke in non-cardiac surgical patients [33]. A further reason adding to perioperative stroke might be a disturbed cerebral autoregulation [34]. Finally—according to the NeuroVISION trial—silent strokes may primarily increase the risk for POCD [31].

2.6 Convulsive status epilepticus (CSE) and non-convulsive status epilepticus (NCSE)

CSE and NCSE have a little higher prevalence in general surgical patients than previously assumed (1–10%). During postoperative intensive care, the prevalence of NCSE further increases up to 30% [35]. Primary predisposing risk factors are structural brain diseases and impaired brain development. A CSE is defined as seizure lasting >30 minutes—importantly, seizures lasting >5 minutes are rarely self-limiting, requiring adequate treatment [36].

The pathophysiology underlying seizures is based on a disbalance of excitatory and inhibitory neuronal brain activity. As a consequence, brain metabolism, cerebral blood flow, blood glucose and lactate levels increase. Consecutively, an elevated cardiac output, tachycardia, hypertension and elevated central venous pressure occur. These pathophysiological changes may represent a compensation of the body potentially protecting the brain for 30–60 minutes. Afterwards, cerebral autoregulation is impaired—leading to cerebral hypoxia, hypoglycaemia, elevated intracranial pressure (ICP) and cerebral oedema. Finally, electrolyte imbalance, metabolic acidosis, disseminated intravascular coagulation and rhabdomyolysis may induce a multi-organ failure [36]. These pathophysiological changes likely apply to NCSE—typically proceeding slower [36, 37].

To prevent perioperative seizures, it is key continuing anti-epileptic medication. While most anaesthetics do not interfere with anti-epileptic medication, quantifying its plasma level in case of postoperative intensive care is recommended [35].

2.7 Cerebral macroangiopathy

Pathologies of cerebral arteries have significant clinical importance—in particular during anaesthesiologic perioperative patient care. Pre-existing cerebral macroangiopathy including a stroke or TIA, a significant carotid artery stenosis and a cerebral artery aneurysm may require a neurological council and subsequently, in individual patients, further diagnostic imaging such as computed tomography (CT) scan, MRI or transcranial Doppler (TCD) ultrasound. Importantly, a pre-existing peripheral artery occlusive disease (PAOD) is regularly combined with an occlusive cerebrovascular disease—potentially significantly affecting cerebral circulation. Among PAOD surgical patients with occlusive cerebrovascular disease, up to 14% have carotid artery stenosis >70% [3]. Hence, a preoperative carotid ultrasound may be a beneficial diagnostic tool to indicate a necessary cerebral revascularisation [38].

Currently, cerebral revascularisation—performed either surgically or by endovascular techniques—is usually done postoperatively as long-term prevention of stroke. Therefore, optimising cardiac output and maintaining adequate cerebral perfusion pressure (CPP) seem crucial. Considering patients with significant atherosclerosis, statins and beta-blockers should be perioperatively applied continuously, and the application of acetylsalicylic acid should be interrupted as short as possible. In addition, blood pressure levels should be targeted according to the guidelines on non-cardiac surgery provided by the European Society of Cardiology (ESC) and the European Society of Anaesthesiology (ESA) (**Table 1**) [3]. Finally, perioperative monitoring may be extended by invasive blood pressure monitoring and transoesophageal echo estimating stroke volume.

2.8 Cerebral microangiopathy and Alzheimer's disease (AD)

Cerebral microangiopathies—diseases of the terminal vessels—potentially impair significantly cerebral microcirculation and play a key role in the pathophysiology of perioperative neuropsychiatric morbidities. Cerebral microangiopathy primarily includes subcortical arteriosclerotic encephalopathy (Binswanger's disease), cerebral amyloid angiopathy and inflammatory-based microangiopathies [39].

Binswanger's disease can be clinically characterised by persistent hypertension and systemic vascular disease, acute strokes, subacute accumulation of focal neurologic symptoms with signs over weeks to months, long plateau periods, lengthy clinical course, dementia, prominent motor signs or pseudobulbar palsy and hydrocephalus. Pathologically, cerebrovascular atherosclerosis of small vessels, a diffuse white matter loss combined with gliosis and lacunar infarcts, can be detected. According to the findings of neuroimaging studies using MRI and CT scans, the term white matter disease has been established [39–41]. While it has been hypothesised that white matter hyperintensities (WMH) may result from degenerative or demyelinating processes, atherosclerotic vascular changes seem to be crucial for the progression of WMH [42].

Risk factors for Binswanger's disease include in particular hypertension, atrial fibrillation and a high patient age [39, 42]. Accordingly, early treatment of hypertension may have a protective effect. However, hypotension (generally, orthostatically, nightly and postprandially) seems to be an additional risk factor. Therefore, blood pressure adjustment to a high-normal range (i.e. systolic blood pressure 135–150 mmHg) is currently recommended [43].

Recommendations	Class of recommendation	Level of evidence
Preoperative carotid artery and cerebral imaging are recommended in patients with a history of TIA or stroke in the preceding 6 months.	I	C
Preoperative, routine carotid artery imaging may be considered in patients undergoing vascular surgery.	IIb	C
Whenever possible, continuation of anti-platelet and statin therapies should be considered throughout the perioperative phase in patients with carotid artery disease.	IIa	C
For patients with carotid artery disease undergoing non-cardiac surgery, the same indications for carotid revascularisation should apply as for the general population.	IIa	C
Preoperative routine carotid artery imaging is not recommended in patients undergoing non-vascular surgery.	III	C

Table 1.
Recommendations on patients with suspected or established carotid artery disease according to the guidelines on non-cardiac surgery provided by the European Society of Cardiology (ESC) and the European Society of Anaesthesiology (ESA).

According to the current concept of mixed dementia, Binswanger's disease promotes AD in the elderly population [44]. Pathophysiologically, AD onset is based on the accumulation of amyloid β inducing hyperphosphorylation of protein tau, leading to neurofibrillary tangles. Heritable factors play a key role in 60–80% of AD patients—more than 40 AD-associated genetic risk loci have already been identified, of which apolipoprotein E alleles have the strongest impact. Positron emission tomography scans and plasma assays may be used to detect amyloid β and phosphorylated tau. Current research further suggests that specific lifestyle factors may contribute to a positive outcome in AD patients. Prospectively, potentially beneficial medical treatment includes anti-amyloid β, anti-tau and anti-inflammatory strategies [45]. Finally, AD (60%) and Binswanger's disease (20%) are the major causes of brain failure in the elderly population [40].

2.9 Cerebral autoregulation dysfunction

Cerebral autoregulation describes the physiological adaption of the cross-section of cerebral arterial vessels to the CPP [46]—thereby enabling a constant cerebral perfusion within a particular range of systemic blood pressure. Deceeding the lower limit of cerebral autoregulation (LLA) decreases cerebral perfusion, potentially impairing cerebral function and resulting in symptoms like seizures and neurocognitive dysfunction. In contrast, exceeding the upper limit of cerebral autoregulation (ULA) subsequently leads to cerebral hyperperfusion, potentially impairing the BBB with consecutive vasogenic cerebral oedema. Generally, cerebral autoregulation is probably controlled by myogenic and endothelial cerebrovascular factors and by metabolic mechanisms [47].

Since the Kety-Schmidt technique has been established in 1948, static cerebral autoregulation could be measured—describing the relationship between mean arterial pressure (MAP) and CPP during a steady-state MAP. Subsequently, Rune Aaslid has established TCD ultrasound in 1982, which had a key impact on measuring dynamic cerebral autoregulation—describing the MAP-CPP relationship during a non-steady-state MAP by his landmark study in 1989 [48]. Since systemic blood pressure slightly varies continuously (e.g. influenced by breathing or physiologically), nowadays, using dynamic cerebral autoregulation is paramount [49].

According to current knowledge, cerebral autoregulation functions correctly within a smaller range of systemic arterial blood pressure than previously assumed [46]—which has been firstly shown in 1997 and later confirmed (**Figure 2**) [47, 49]. Both the LLA seems to vary individually within 40–90 mmHg and the shape of the LLA may strongly vary. In addition, the plateau of the cerebral autoregulation curve (**Figure 2**) may be rather small—about 20 mmHg [47]. Importantly, various patients can probably better compensate exceeding the ULA than deceeding the LLA [49]. Accordingly, adjusting blood pressure individually during perioperative anaesthesiologic patient care seems to play a key role [47].

Dynamic cerebral autoregulation can be studied on one side by time domain analysis: by measuring the degree of correlation between blood pressure and various cerebral output signals, the Pearson correlation coefficient is calculated. While a positive correlation coefficient reflects synchrony between the two signals—suggesting an impaired cerebral autoregulation—a negative or near-zero correlation coefficient implies a physiological adaption to blood pressure changes, indicating an intact cerebral autoregulation. A further measuring approach is based on more complex analyses of time-frequency domains [50]. Currently, dynamic cerebral autoregulation

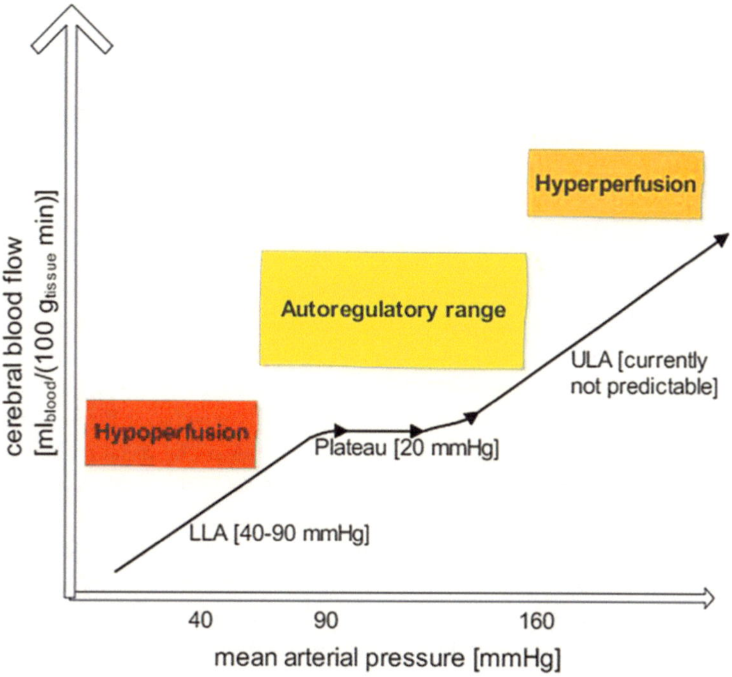

Figure 2.
Adjusted curve of cerebral autoregulation. Both the lower limit (LLA) and upper limit (ULA) of cerebral autoregulation vary significantly between individual surgical patients.

is usually determined by two input signals—invasive or non-invasive arterial blood pressure combined with cerebral blood flow (e.g. estimated by TCD ultrasound), ICP or regional oxygen saturation (rSO_2) of the brain estimated by near-infrared spectroscopy (NIRS) [51].

According to current research, cerebral autoregulation may be in particular impaired in elderly patients (e.g. based on micro- or macroangiopathy, diabetes and dementia) and perioperatively (e.g. based on mechanical ventilation, delirium, SIRS and dialysis)—indicating that a perioperative bedside monitoring might be beneficial [47]. In line with an international consensus paper regarding perioperative intensive care, monitoring of cerebral autoregulation is especially recommended for individually selected neurocritical care patients [52]. Currently, intraoperative monitoring of cerebral autoregulation cannot be routinely performed; however, it can be done in clinical research.

2.10 Limited cognitive reserve (CR)

CR is the capacity of the brain to compensate for a varying range of cerebral injuries without functional cerebral impairment—this concept has been firstly described at the end of the 80s [53]. CR is primarily based on good cerebral functionality and brain plasticity, which enables the brain to make neurostructural changes for adaption to potential impairments.

Since CR represents a theoretical concept, it is usually measured by proxy variables including general lifetime experiences, educational and occupational attainment, intelligence, lifestyle (e.g. social, physical and cognitive activities), socioeconomic status and early life experiences (e.g. perinatal and postnatal factors such as childhood intelligence). In addition, biomarker studies examining amyloid and tau protein may be used. The concept of CR—potentially playing a significant role in age-related cognitive dysfunction based on describing individual differences in susceptibility to cognitive, functional or clinical decline—may be applicable to multiple neuropsychiatric morbidities including AD, macro- and microangiopathy, delirium and other [54, 55]. Since only about 50% of inter-individual variability in cognitive dysfunction is based on the most common age-related neuropathology, such as AD, various neurodegenerative and cerebrovascular factors may significantly add to the pathophysiology underlying cognitive dysfunction in the growing elderly population [56]. Finally, there is strong evidence that a high level of CR proxy variables is associated with a lower risk of mild cognitive dysfunction and dementia in the elderly [54].

Current research suggests that specific features such as education, genetic factors, physical activity, older age at retirement and wealth increase CR, allowing individuals being more resilient by influencing the efficiency, capacity or flexibility of brain networks, cerebral vasculature, cerebral metabolism and neurochemical transmission—and in this way better coping with age-related brain diseases. On the contrary, specific features including smoking, obesity, genetics, an early onset or elevated rate of cerebral pathology, early life hardship (e.g. the death of a parent) and prenatal factors (e.g. small birth weight) may decrease CR—thus depressing the threshold of cerebral compensation of negative effects on brain health [54, 57–60]. Latest research indicates that some cerebral mechanisms elevating the threshold at which cerebral compensation works seem to be similar to cerebral mechanisms in young adults managing highly challenging cognitive and behavioural tasks. Moreover, less age-related anatomic cerebral changes like brain atrophy, limited task-related networks and WMH, together with a low cerebral pathology accumulation over time, may increase CR [61]. Finally, in some elderly individuals, the anatomic or physiological cerebral processes involved in cognition may improve above current levels, which at least may attenuate typical age-related brain changes [54, 62].

According to Stern's theory, a high level of CR may have a beneficial influence on perioperative neuropsychiatric patient outcome in two ways—by a higher preoperative level of cognitive performance and by a delayed onset of an induced perioperative cognitive decline. However, since a high level of CR may be associated with a better compensation of cerebral pathology accumulation, a high level of CR may be paradoxically associated with a faster rate of perioperative cognitive decline once cerebral injuries are severe enough to impair cognitive function [57]. This points out the potential benefits of future preoperative baseline and perioperative follow-up diagnosis of CR.

3. Identifying perioperative patients with pre-existing neuropsychiatric morbidities

3.1 Specific methods to identify pre-existing neuropsychiatric morbidities

Identifying neuropsychiatric morbidities is primarily based on exploring the central nervous system (CNS) and surrounding structures including the vasculature of the CNS and the peripheral nervous system. Related to perioperative anaesthesiologic patient care, the detection of pre-existing neuropsychiatric morbidities is of major importance. In particular, exploring exactly the preoperative anamnesis and a detailed clinical examination, ideally including psychometric test batteries should be performed. In addition, neuroimaging tools including an ultrasound of the carotid arteries, TCD ultrasound, CT scan, MRI, NIRS and EEG may be useful in individual patients.

3.2 Preoperative anamnesis

As part of the preoperative anamnesis neuropsychiatric morbidities including seizures, paralysis and sensibility disorders potentially based on a pre-existing stroke or TIA, dementia, cerebral macro- or microangiopathy, depression, anxiety disorders and more subtle cerebral impairments such as mild cognitive dysfunction should be explored. Since cerebral macro- and microangiopathy elevate the risk for perioperative neuropsychiatric disorders including disturbed cerebral autoregulation, and may be associated with potentially existing angiopathies such as coronary heart disease and PAOD and their underlying risk factors—hypertension, hypercholesterolaemia, diabetes and cigarette smoking—these facts should be considered [63]. A drug-abusing behaviour (e.g. alcohol, nicotine, drug and medical abuse) should be further explored. Finally, asking for family anamnesis may allow for detecting preoperative neurological morbidities which are partly associated with genes (e.g. multiple sclerosis (MS), dementia, seizures, migraine and stroke).

3.3 Neuropsychiatric testing and the postoperative quality of recovery scale (PostopQRS)

The Framingham Heart Study discovered that cognitive dysfunction is associated with higher patient morbidity and mortality [63]. This finding might be applicable to perioperative anaesthesiologic patient care, as suggested by research investigating non-cardiac surgical patients [64], which is why a preoperative evaluation of cognitive function seems to be beneficial. However, a complete neuropsychiatric examination including multiple psychometric tests would last about 60–120 minutes, and the specific types of tests usually vary depending on the specific hospital. The latter along with inconclusive research results underpin the difficulty of testing for cognitive dysfunction during the perioperative period. In addition, perioperative neuropsychiatric testing may be further complicated by various other factors (e.g. restless surroundings, pain and sleep disturbances).

The PostopQRS is a simple web-based digital tool to assess clinical outcomes in surgical patients related to the quality of postoperative recovery. Accordingly, the main domains of postoperative recovery consisting of physiologic, nociceptive, functional, cognitive and emotional recovery are assessed over time. The development of the PostopQRS was started in 2007 by an international research group [65]. Subsequently, a refinement was performed in accordance with sector good practices such as the United States Food and Drug Administration (FDA) guidance. Ongoing developments have further suggested that the PostopQRS allows for analysing normal cognitive performance variability, discriminating changes between patient groups and detecting cognitive decline prior to surgery. In addition, the PostopQRS has been validated for surgical patients ≥6 years, can be completed within 5–6 minutes and can also be done using a pen and paper completion questionnaire [65–67].

Since the quality of life after patient discharge from the hospital is of crucial importance, further simple tools evaluating the quality of recovery after major surgeries appropriate for clinical practice such as the PostopQRS may gain in importance in the future [67, 68].

3.4 Screening for dementia by psychometric tests

Psychometric tests can be used to screen for specific stages of dementia, which plays an important role in perioperative patient care. In 1975, the

Mini-Mental-Status-Exam (MMSE) has been established as clinical tool allowing for grading perioperative cognitive dysfunction. Using MMSE, cognitive function is assessed by 30 tasks examining temporal and spatial orientation, retentiveness, memory capability, attention, language and speech comprehension, reading and writing capability, drawing and calculating. Each successfully resolved task gives one point and accordingly achievable a maximum score of 30 points. Typically, a score < 25 represents a mild cognitive impairment (MCI), a score < 20 a moderate cognitive impairment and a score < 10 a severe cognitive impairment or dementia—however, these cut-off points may not be appropriate for each patient [69, 70].

Although the MMSE can be used as an efficient clinical psychometric test for both grading cognitive impairment and detecting dementia perioperatively, sensitivity and specificity may be impaired by various features including patient age, individual education, reduced visual and hearing performance, tremors, difficulties in reading, a preceding stroke or TIA, nervousness, pain and the hospital environment. Hence, another psychometric test, the Montreal Cognitive Assessment (MoCA), has been developed, which might be superior to the MMSE—in particular in detecting MCI [70]. One more test, the Functional Assessment Staging Test (FAST) allowing for grading AD (1–7f) has been developed in 1984 [71, 72].

Finally, since, for one thing, MCI and dementia increase related to a growing elderly population and, on the other hand, improved cognitive abilities can be observed in individual elderly people, psychometric tests should be regularly updated to stay accurate in clinical practice [73].

3.5 Neuroimaging using magnetic resonance imaging (MRI) and computed tomography (CT) scan

Modern MRI algorithms have significantly contributed to current knowledge about perioperative neuropsychiatric morbidities, in particular concerning impaired perfusion of the white matter of the brain [41]. The term subcortical vascular dementia incorporates lacunar strokes, Binswanger's disease and vascular dementia. Lacunar strokes represent small-sized infarcts based on the occlusion of small cerebral arteries penetrating the basal ganglia, the brain stem and the white matter—potentially associated with cerebral microangiopathy based on hypertension. Binswanger's disease is represented as WMH using MRI, which shows bilaterally spotted brain areas diffusely localised in the white matter. In the T2 weighted image—one of the basic pulse sequences of MRI highlighting differences in the T2 relaxation time of tissues—WMH can be displayed. These WMH are probably caused by reduced perfusion of the white matter, while the grey matter is typically normally perfused [74]. Histopathologically, a gliosis, a demyelination and a loss of neuronal axons can be seen. Currently, it remains unclear whether vascular dementia is primarily based on a disturbed BBB or on chronic hypoperfusion inducing an inflammatory brain response—potentially depending on microangiopathy. MRI studies suggest that WMH may be a predictor for POCD onset [75]. The early clinical sign of a gait disorder with a tendency to fall can be seen in both vascular dementia and Binswanger's disease.

Diffusion tensor imaging (DTI)—an MRI technique that uses anisotropic diffusion to estimate the white matter organisation of the brain—may allow for detecting early stages of cerebral injuries. In particular, pathological changes in the white matter can be precisely displayed, which can be used in the diagnosis of early strokes within the white matter. Further applications include the detection of an early onset of AD, schizophrenia, focal cortical dysplasia, MS including plaque assessment, early identification of peripheral nerve pathology and presurgical planning. Finally, fibre tractography is a three-dimensional reconstruction technique based on DTI to assess white matter tracts [76].

CT scans are less exact than modern MRI techniques; however, they are much more widely available. In clinical practice, performing a perioperative CT scan is quite easier than an MRI—in particular with critically ill patients. Therefore, CT scans are a good option to detect cerebral bleeding, while ischaemic strokes are later and less precisely seen on a CT scan than on MRI. Furthermore, computed tomography angiography (CTA)—using an injection of a contrast media into a venous blood vessel—allows for detecting blood vessel diseases like aneurysms, stenoses and occlusions. Both CT scans and MRI can beneficially support individual perioperative patient care.

3.6 Non-invasive screening tools for neuropsychiatric morbidities

Modern non-invasive screening tools to detect neuropsychiatric morbidities include measuring the intima-media thickness (IMT), TCD ultrasound, NIRS and processed EEG (pEEG).

Assessing the IMT allows for detecting subclinical atherosclerosis and should be done in every asymptomatic adult perioperative patient having a moderate risk for cardiovascular disease and in hypertensive patients. An IMT > 0.9 mm according to the ESC or over the 75th percentile according to the American Society of Echocardiography (ASE) is considered as pathological. A carotid artery ultrasound scan is the method of choice for measuring the IMT. However, the results of IMT may be biased by different factors including the present haemodynamic, blood pressure levels and the stretching of cerebral vessels [77].

Since 1982, intracerebral vessels can be evaluated by TCD ultrasound [48]. Currently, an advanced, multifrequency pulsed TCD ultrasound is the device of choice to investigate in particular both middle cerebral arteries through the temporal acoustic window. The cerebral blood flow velocity (CBFV) can be continuously recorded, and a reduced CBFV can potentially indicate that a reduced cerebral perfusion is present. However, a wide range of the mean CBFV (38–86 cm/s) of the middle cerebral artery—which further depends on the angle of the transducers' position—has to be considered. Calculating the pulsatility index (PI [PI = (Systolic velocity – diastolic velocity)/mean velocity]) allows for examining cerebrovascular resistance. A PI >1 indicates an elevated vascular resistance typically combined with reduced vascular compliance—which is often based on arterial hypertension and other cardiovascular risk factors [78].

According to current literature, a high patient age is associated with a reduced CBFV and an elevated PI [79]. TCD ultrasound enables the detection of various cerebrovascular pathologies in real time including cerebral ischaemia [78]. Notably, reduced cerebral perfusion is suggested to be associated with higher cardiovascular and non-cardiovascular mortality [2].

A further application of TCD ultrasound is measuring dynamic cerebral autoregulation using CBFV and MAP as input signals [48]. This approach may optimise blood pressure adjustment perioperatively, which may be especially important since a disturbed cerebral autoregulation commonly impairs cerebral perfusion. Importantly, dynamic cerebral autoregulation may be frequently impaired in the elderly population and in multiple neuropsychiatric and other morbidities including MCI, AD, sepsis, hypothermia, anaemia, hypercapnia, obstructive sleep apnoea and acute respiratory distress syndrome—which all may occur during perioperative patient care

[78]. In addition, modern multifrequency TCD devices allow for quantifying cerebral microemboli and further differentiate microemboli into gaseous or solid ones by TCD software algorithms [80]. Cerebral microemboli are for example detectable distal of a stent or during postoperative intensive care if patients are treated with extracorporeal circuits such as dialysis or ECMO—especially venoarterial ECMO may induce a high number of cerebral microemboli (**Figure 1**) [10]. According to current research, the clinical consequences of cerebral microemboli remain unclear—suggesting that they could play a role in the pathophysiology of more subtle neuropsychiatric morbidities like POCD and MCI [18, 81].

Currently, TCD ultrasound is routinely performed in neurocritical care patients, while in other critically ill patients, it is rarely done during the perioperative period. The main limitation of TCD ultrasound is an inadequate temporal acoustic window (10–15%) [78].

NIRS uses near-infrared light (wavelength of 700–900 nm) being able to penetrate living tissue. The technical principle is based on the fact that the ratio of infrared light absorbed to that scattered by haemoglobin changes depending on the degree of haemoglobin binding with oxygen. NIRS calculates this rate of change and the change in oxygenated haemoglobin concentration. These changes in rSO_2 correlate with the regional cerebral oxygenation, estimating roughly regional cerebral blood flow. To indicate regional cerebral oxygenation, the tissue oxygen index (TOI; standard value = 50%) is calculated. NIRS-based analyses may indicate a reduced regional cerebral perfusion since rSO_2 accordingly decreases, which is displayed as a lower level of TOI—a TOI < 35% indicates potential tissue damage based on cerebral ischaemia. However, rSO_2 depends additionally on other features such as body temperature and present haemoglobin values. Nonetheless, NIRS provides an easily applicable tool to monitor rSO_2 during the perioperative period [82].

Continuous pEEG monitoring is technically complex and rather prone to artefacts. During the last decades, different pEEG methods have been developed such as the bispectral index (BIS) and Narcotrend, to reduce, in particular, intraoperative awareness. In addition, pEEG monitoring should help anaesthesiologists in both targeting an optimised depth of anaesthesia and shortening the anaesthetic recovery phase [83]. The prevalence of intraoperative awareness is about 0.5–2/1000 patients. After reviewing the available literature, it remains unclear whether pEEG monitoring significantly reduces intraoperative awareness. In line with current research, pEEG-guided TIVA based on propofol may reduce intraoperative awareness, while a minimum alveolar concentration (MAC)-guided volatile anaesthesia may be equally effective [84–86]. Accordingly, pEEG-guided anaesthesia may be a beneficial tool but cannot replace the intraoperative clinical evaluation of the depth of anaesthesia (e.g. heart frequency, blood pressure levels, ventilation patterns, sweating and slight body movements) [86]. Finally, current research may show whether pEEG monitoring can be beneficially used during postoperative patient care—in particular in critically ill patients.

4. Treatment recommendations for perioperative anaesthesiologic care of non-cardiac surgical patients with neuropsychiatric morbidities

4.1 Perioperative hypotension and cerebral hypoxia

Multiple studies have shown that intraoperative hypotension is associated with increased general organ impairment, which may be also applicable to the brain [87].

Prolonged intraoperative hypotension during major surgeries may elevate the risk for postoperative stroke—however, research has produced inconclusive data [33, 87, 88]. In line with current knowledge, the accumulation of intraoperative hypotensive periods giving the complete time of intraoperative hypotension seems to be of significant clinical importance, since clinical practice has shown that multiple hypotensive periods during intraoperative anaesthesia can frequently happen. Accordingly, increasing total hypotensive periods may elevate in non-cardiac surgical patients the risk for postoperative cerebral impairment and may increase the postoperative mortality in elderly patients, while short periods of the lowest acceptable intraoperative blood pressures are suggested to be better tolerated [89].

Currently, it can be recommended to target blood pressure adjustment intraoperatively—applicable to both adults and infants—in relation to baseline levels present in a calm preoperative waking state within a range of ±20% (maximally ±30%), concerning additionally the evidence suggesting that a MAP threshold <55–60 mmHg is frequently associated with organ injury [90, 91]. Importantly, this threshold may be unsafe for individual patients including those with coronary artery or cerebrovascular disease potentially requiring a significantly higher MAP [91]. Accordingly, perioperative blood pressure adjustment should be performed based on individual patient demand, since an optimised blood pressure is crucial for sufficient cerebral oxygenation. Similar to the potential harm of intraoperative accumulation of hypotensive periods [89], an accumulation of diffuse cerebral hypoxia impairs postoperative recovery in patients undergoing major general surgeries [92]. Considering clinical practice, in non-cardiac surgical patients, an intermittent cerebral hypoxia, can occur in up to one out of four patients and is associated with POCD and a longer hospital stay—in particular in the elderly patient population [93].

4.2 Triple-low

The term triple-low has been established by Sessler's research group in 2012 and refers to a low BIS (<45), a low MAP (<75 mmHg) and a low MAC (<0.8) during surgery—which has been shown being associated with an increased risk for patient mortality [94].

Since an association between a BIS <45 and postoperative mortality has been reported in non-cardiac surgical patients, the depth of anaesthesia has been discussed by many clinicians to be causally related to this finding [94]. However, aside from inducing hypotension, there is currently no evidence that anaesthetic agents are directly toxic to the brain or other organs. In addition, one would expect a decreased mortality in surgical patients undergoing regional instead of general anaesthesia—which could not be shown according to current research [91]. Although a cumulative time of BIS <45 in cardiac surgery has been related to postoperative patient mortality, a BIS <45 was paradoxically not associated with an increased volatile anaesthetic exposure. Even more surprisingly, an increased volatile anaesthetic exposure was not associated with patient mortality [95]. Hence, the occasional dissociation between a low BIS and a high volatile anaesthetic concentration remains to be elucidated.

Sessler's large study including a non-cardiac surgical population showed that triple-low was highly predictive of postoperative death [94]. However, regarding controversies in science, some studies did not support this association [91]. Accordingly, Goodman's study group recommended a standard approach for judging research reproducibility [96]. The main reason for conflicting study results is suggested to be the BIS algorithm. While both blood pressure and volatile anaesthetic concentrations can be measured using quantifiable units such as mmHg and kPa, allowing for a reliable comparison between patients, BIS algorithm includes a concept of a linear scale from 100 to 0, reflecting the depth of anaesthesia. This scale concept is further not supported by a biological rationale, and in addition, BIS algorithm has been regularly revised over time—which probably leads to a lack of reliable patient comparison. Furthermore, the BIS scale does not decrease consistently with the depth of anaesthesia and sometimes paradoxically increases though volatile anaesthetic concentration increases [97]. In addition, aside from being vulnerable to artefacts (e.g. extracranial electrical activity), the sole application of neuromuscular blocking agents significantly decreases BIS [98]. Hence, a low BIS might not be a reliable parameter within the triple-low concept to predict patient mortality, while other intraoperative EEG features like electrical suppression are related to impaired postoperative outcome [91].

Finally, in line with current knowledge, triple-low events can significantly predict a higher postoperative mortality rate but in particular a low BIS may be not related to the underlying causality [91, 99].

4.3 The 2-hit model of cerebral impairment

In line with current knowledge, an individually adapted perioperative anaesthesiologic patient care—including an optimised intraoperative anaesthesia—seems to be crucial for postoperative patient outcome [87, 91]. The 2-hit model of

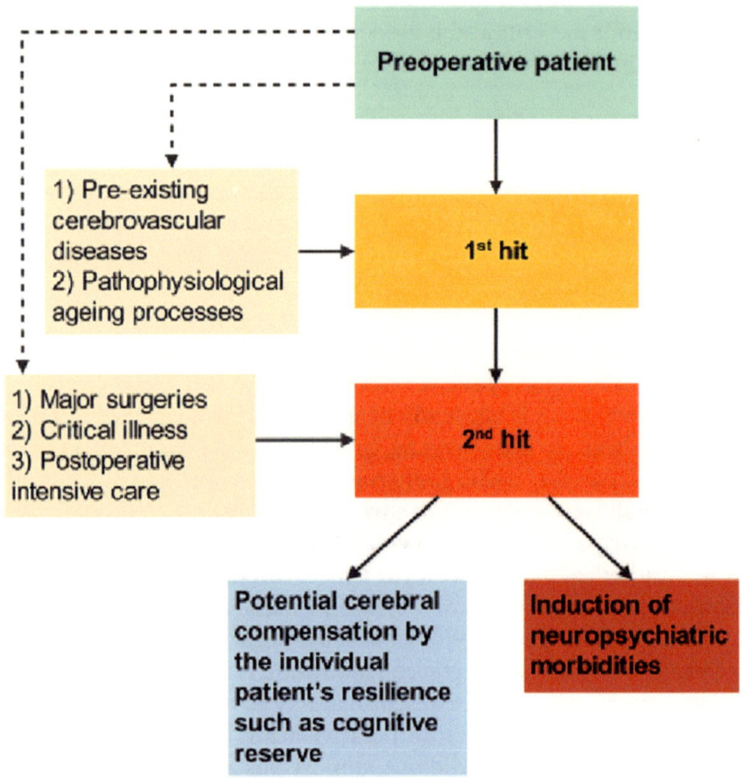

Figure 3.
The 2-hit model of cerebral impairment. While the first hit may be well compensated by individual elderly patients, the second hit seems being much more difficult to be compensated.

perioperative cerebral impairment describes a hypothetical theory based on current research [39, 89, 99] similar to a suggested 2-hit model of PTSD [100]. In particular, pre-existing cerebrovascular diseases (i.e. macro- and microangiopathy) together with a pathophysiological ageing process may lead to a first cerebral impairment (first hit) [39], which may be well compensated by individual elderly patients [41]. Subsequently, perioperative surgical and anaesthesiologic patient care may induce a second cerebral impairment (second hit), which seems to be much more difficult to compensate by the patient—particularly in cases of major surgeries, critical illness and postoperative intensive care [8, 18].

Depending on the severity of the first and second hit, considering individual patients' resilience such as CR or patient age, neuropsychiatric morbidities may be induced (**Figure 3**). Concerning postoperative patient outcome, it is of major importance to significantly reduce the second hit by individually optimised perioperative anaesthesiologic patient care [91].

5. Conclusions

In summary, neuropsychiatric morbidities play a significant role in perioperative anaesthesiologic patient care—including preoperative assessment, intraoperative general or regional anaesthesia and postoperative intensive care in case of critical illness or major surgeries—due to their associated impaired postoperative quality of life and their affection of overall patient outcome. Therefore, a key factor is the maintenance of an individual's patient homeostasis. Accordingly, this concept includes that baseline levels (e.g. blood pressure, heart frequency and specific blood values such as natrium and CO_2) the individual patient has been getting used to potentially over the years, should be only adapted within a rather small range (i.e. ± 20%). In case of unknown preoperative baseline levels, the following targets should be aspired to: normotension, normovolaemia, normocapnia, normoxaemia, normothermia and normoglycaemia. Patients at higher risk for neuropsychiatric morbidities may benefit from additional neuromonitoring tools (e.g. NIRS, TCD ultrasound and pEEG-guided anaesthesia). In addition, surgical patients profit from early mobilisation, an optimised pain therapy and an early return to everyday life as soon as possible after surgery. Considering in particular postoperative intensive care and critical illness, these treatment steps should be completed with further individual anaesthesiologic patient care (e.g. early weaning from the respirator or at least targeting spontaneous breathing and a treatment of postoperative delirium in line with current guidelines). Finally, the development of new neuromonitoring techniques will may allow for reducing perioperative neuropsychiatric morbidities in the future.

Acknowledgements

I especially thank *Dr. Klaus Ulrich Klein*, PhD, Associate Professor, MBA and head of the Department of Anaesthesia and Intensive Care of the Sanatorium Hera, a private hospital in Vienna, Austria. He supported me in writing this book chapter by giving important intellectual input and, in addition, as a scientific advisor.

All sources of funding were provided by the Department of General Anaesthesia and Critical Care, Medical University of Vienna, Austria. No external funding was obtained.

Conflict of interest

The author declares no conflict of interest.

Author details

Clemens Kietaibl
Department of General Anaesthesia and Critical Care, Medical University of Vienna, Vienna, Austria

*Address all correspondence to: clemens.kietaibl@meduniwien.ac.at

References

[1] Fleisher LA, Fleischmann KE, Auerbach AD, Barnason SA, Beckman JA, Bozkurt B, et al. 2014 ACC/AHA guideline on perioperative cardiovascular evaluation and management of patients undergoing noncardiac surgery: A report of the American College of Cardiology/ American Heart Association Task Force on Practice Guidelines. Circulation. 2014;**130**:e278-e333. DOI: 10.1161/ CIR.0000000000000106

[2] Sabayan B, van der Grond J, Westendorp RG, Jukema JW, Ford I, Buckley BM, et al. Total cerebral blood flow and mortality in old age: A 12-year follow-up study. Neurology. 2013;**81**:1922-1929. DOI: 10.1212/01. wnl.0000436618.48402.da

[3] Kristensen SD, Knuuti J, Saraste A, Anker S, Botker HE, Hert SD, et al. 2014 ESC/ESA guidelines on non-cardiac surgery: Cardiovascular assessment and management: The Joint Task Force on non-cardiac surgery: Cardiovascular assessment and management of the European Society of Cardiology (ESC) and the European Society of Anaesthesiology (ESA). European Heart Journal. 2014;**35**:2383-2431. DOI: 10.1093/eurheartj/ehu282

[4] Kehlet H, Jensen TS, Woolf CJ. Persistent postsurgical pain: Risk factors and prevention. Lancet. 2006;**367**:1618-1625. DOI: 10.1016/ S0140-6736(06)68700-X

[5] Moyce Z, Rodseth RN, Biccard BM. The efficacy of peri-operative interventions to decrease postoperative delirium in non-cardiac surgery: A systematic review and meta-analysis. Anaesthesia. 2014;**69**:259-269. DOI: 10.1111/anae.12539

[6] Girard TD, Pandharipande PP, Ely EW. Delirium in the intensive care unit. Critical Care. 2008;**12**(Suppl. 3):S3. DOI: 10.1186/cc6149

[7] Rudolph JL, Marcantonio ER. Review articles: Postoperative delirium: Acute change with long-term implications. Anesthesia and Analgesia. 2011;**112**:1202-1211. DOI: 10.1213/ ANE.0b013e3182147f6d

[8] Zaal IJ, Devlin JW, Peelen LM, Slooter AJ. A systematic review of risk factors for delirium in the ICU. Critical Care Medicine. 2015;**43**:40-47. DOI: 10.1097/CCM.0000000000000625

[9] Lee HB, Mears SC, Rosenberg PB, Leoutsakos JM, Gottschalk A, Sieber FE. Predisposing factors for postoperative delirium after hip fracture repair in individuals with and without dementia. Journal of the American Geriatrics Society. 2011;**59**:2306-2313. DOI: 10.1111/j.1532-5415.2011.03725.x

[10] Kietaibl C, Horvat Menih I, Engel A, Ullrich R, Klein KU, Erdoes G. Cerebral microemboli during extracorporeal life support: A single-centre cohort study. European Journal of Cardio-Thoracic Surgery. 2021;**61**:172-179. DOI: 10.1093/ ejcts/ezab353

[11] Piva S, McCreadie VA, Latronico N. Neuroinflammation in sepsis: Sepsis associated delirium. Cardiovascular & Hematological Disorders Drug Targets. 2015;**15**:10-18. DOI: 10.2174/1871529x 15666150108112452

[12] Wachtendorf LJ, Azimaraghi O, Santer P, Linhardt FC, Blank M, Suleiman A, et al. Association between intraoperative arterial hypotension and postoperative delirium after noncardiac

surgery: A retrospective multicenter cohort study. Anesthesia and Analgesia. 2022;**134**:822-833. DOI: 10.1213/ANE.0000000000005739

[13] Mashour GA, Woodrum DT, Avidan MS. Neurological complications of surgery and anaesthesia. British Journal of Anaesthesia. 2015;**114**:194-203. DOI: 10.1093/bja/aeu296

[14] Khanna AK, Shaw AD, Stapelfeldt WH, Boero IJ, Chen Q, Stevens M, et al. Postoperative hypotension and adverse clinical outcomes in patients without intraoperative hypotension, after noncardiac surgery. Anesthesia & Analgesia. 2021;**132**:1410-1420. DOI: 10.1213/ANE.0000000000005374

[15] Smischney NJ, Shaw AD, Stapelfeldt WH, Boero IJ, Chen Q, Stevens M, et al. Postoperative hypotension in patients discharged to the intensive care unit after non-cardiac surgery is associated with adverse clinical outcomes. Critical Care. 2020;**24**:682. DOI: 10.1186/s13054-020-03412-5

[16] Newman S, Stygall J, Hirani S, Shaefi S, Maze M. Postoperative cognitive dysfunction after noncardiac surgery: A systematic review. Anesthesiology. 2007;**106**:572-590. DOI: 10.1097/00000542-200703000-00023

[17] Travica N, Lotfaliany M, Marriott A, Safavynia SA, Lane MM, Gray L, et al. Peri-operative risk factors associated with post-operative cognitive dysfunction (POCD): An umbrella review of Meta-analyses of observational studies. Journal of Clinical Medicine. 2023;**12**:1610. DOI: 10.3390/jcm12041610

[18] Silbert BS, Evered LA, Scott DA, Rahardja S, Gerraty RP, Choong PF. Review of transcranial Doppler ultrasound to detect microemboli during orthopedic surgery. AJNR. American Journal of Neuroradiology. 2014;**35**:1858-1863. DOI: 10.3174/ajnr.A3688

[19] Parker AM, Sricharoenchai T, Raparla S, Schneck KW, Bienvenu OJ, Needham DM. Posttraumatic stress disorder in critical illness survivors: A meta analysis. Critical Care Medicine. 2015;**43**:1121-1129. DOI: 10.1097/CCM.0000000000000882

[20] Wofford K, Hertzberg M, VacchianoC.Theperioperativeimplications of posttraumatic stress disorder. AANA Journal. 2012;**80**:463-470 PMID: 23409641

[21] Drews T, Franck M, Radtke FM, Weiss B, Krampe H, Brockhaus WR, et al. Postoperative delirium is an independent risk factor for posttraumatic stress disorder in the elderly patient: A prospective observational study. European Journal of Anaesthesiology. 2015;**32**:147-151. DOI: 10.1097/EJA.0000000000000107

[22] Mashour GA. Posttraumatic stress disorder after intraoperative awareness and high-risk surgery. Anesthesia and Analgesia. 2010;**110**:668-670. DOI: 10.1213/ANE.0b013e3181c35926

[23] Wintermann GB, Brunkhorst FM, Petrowski K, Strauss B, Oehmichen F, Pohl M, et al. Stress disorders following prolonged critical illness in survivors of severe sepsis. Critical Care Medicine. 2015;**43**:1213-1222. DOI: 10.1097/CCM.0000000000000936

[24] Regier DA, Kuhl EA, Kupfer DJ. The DSM-5: Classification and criteria changes. World Psychiatry. 2013;**12**:92-98. DOI: 10.1002/wps.20050

[25] Aceto P, Perilli V, Lai C, Sacco T, Ancona P, Gasperin E, et al. Update

on post-traumatic stress syndrome after anesthesia. European Review for Medical and Pharmacological Sciences. 2013;**17**:1730-1737 PMID: 23852895

[26] O'Doherty DC, Chitty KM, Saddiqui S, Bennett MR, Lagopoulos J. A systematic review and meta-analysis of magnetic resonance imaging measurement of structural volumes in posttraumatic stress disorder. Psychiatry Research. 2015;**232**:1-33. DOI: 10.1016/j.pscychresns.2015.01.002

[27] Roberts MB, Glaspey LJ, Mazzarelli A, Jones CW, Kilgannon HJ, Trzeciak S, et al. Early interventions for the prevention of posttraumatic stress symptoms in survivors of critical illness: A qualitative systematic review. Critical Care Medicine. 2018;**46**:1328-1333. DOI: 10.1097/CCM.0000000000003222

[28] Hori H, Kim Y. Inflammation and post-traumatic stress disorder. Psychiatry and Clinical Neurosciences. 2019;**73**:143-153. DOI: 10.1111/pcn.12820

[29] Mashour GA, Shanks AM, Kheterpal S. Perioperative stroke and associated mortality after noncardiac, nonneurologic surgery. Anesthesiology. 2011;**114**:1289-1296. DOI: 10.1097/ALN.0b013e318216e7f4

[30] Ng JL, Chan MT, Gelb AW. Perioperative stroke in noncardiac, nonneurosurgical surgery. Anesthesiology. 2011;**115**:879-890. DOI: 10.1097/ALN.0b013e31822e9499

[31] Neuro VI. Perioperative covert stroke in patients undergoing non-cardiac surgery (NeuroVISION): A prospective cohort study. Lancet. 2019;**394**:1022-1029. DOI: 10.1016/S0140-6736(19)31795-7

[32] Mashour GA, Moore LE, Lele AV, Robicsek SA, Gelb AW. Perioperative care of patients at high risk for stroke during or after non-cardiac, non-neurologic surgery: Consensus statement from the Society for Neuroscience in Anesthesiology and Critical Care*. Journal of Neurosurgical Anesthesiology. 2014;**26**:273-285. DOI: 10.1097/ANA.0000000000000087

[33] Group PS, Devereaux PJ, Yang H, Yusuf S, Guyatt G, Leslie K, et al. Effects of extended-release metoprolol succinate in patients undergoing non-cardiac surgery (POISE trial): A randomised controlled trial. Lancet. 2008;**371**:1839-1847. DOI: 10.1016/S0140-6736(08)60601-7

[34] Selim M. Perioperative stroke. The New England Journal of Medicine. 2007;**356**:706-713. DOI: 10.1056/NEJMra062668

[35] Perks A, Cheema S, Mohanraj R. Anaesthesia and epilepsy. British Journal of Anaesthesia. 2012;**108**:562-571. DOI: 10.1093/bja/aes027

[36] Lee SK. Diagnosis and treatment of status epilepticus. Journal of Epilepsy Research. 2020;**10**:45-54. DOI: 10.14581/jer.20008

[37] Pollak L, Gandelman-Marton R, Margolin N, Boxer M, Blatt I. Clinical and electroencephalographic findings in acutely ill adults with non-convulsive vs convulsive status epilepticus. Acta Neurologica Scandinavica. 2014;**129**:405-411. DOI: 10.1111/ane.12200

[38] Kaproth-Joslin KA, Bhatt S, Scoutt LM, Rubens DJ. The essentials of extracranial carotid ultrasonographic imaging. Radiologic Clinics of North America. 2014;**52**:1325-1342. DOI: 10.1016/j.rcl.2014.07.010

[39] Group LS. 2001-2011: A decade of the LADIS (Leukoaraiosis and DISability)

study: What have we learned about white matter changes and small-vessel disease? Cerebrovascular Diseases. 2011;**32**:577-588. DOI: 10.1159/000334498

[40] Pantoni L. Cerebral small vessel disease: From pathogenesis and clinical characteristics to therapeutic challenges. Lancet Neurology. 2010;**9**:689-701. DOI: 10.1016/S1474-4422(10)70104-6

[41] Hannawi Y, Vaishnav A, Coskun EP, Gangadhara S, Romero JR. Covert cerebral small vessel disease: Ready for clinical prime time. Journal of the American Heart Association. 2023;**12**:e029891. DOI: 10.1161/JAHA.123.029891

[42] Gottesman RF, Coresh J, Catellier DJ, Sharrett AR, Rose KM, Coker LH, et al. Blood pressure and white-matter disease progression in a biethnic cohort: Atherosclerosis risk in communities (ARIC) study. Stroke. 2010;**41**:3-8. DOI: 10.1161/STROKEAHA.109.566992

[43] Goldberg I, Auriel E, Russell D, Korczyn AD. Microembolism, silent brain infarcts and dementia. Journal of the Neurological Sciences. 2012;**322**:250-253. DOI: 10.1016/j.jns.2012.02.021

[44] Cavalieri M, Schmidt H, Schmidt R. Structural MRI in normal aging and Alzheimer's disease: White and black spots. Neurodegenerative Diseases. 2012;**10**:253-256. DOI: 10.1159/000333120

[45] Scheltens P, De Strooper B, Kivipelto M, Holstege H, Chetelat G, Teunissen CE, et al. Alzheimer's disease. Lancet. 2021;**397**:1577-1590. DOI: 10.1016/S0140-6736(20)32205-4

[46] Lassen NA. Cerebral blood flow and oxygen consumption in man. Physiological Reviews. 1959;**39**:183-238. DOI: 10.1152/physrev.1959.39.2.183

[47] Moerman A, De Hert S. Why and how to assess cerebral autoregulation? Best Practice & Research. Clinical Anaesthesiology. 2019;**33**:211-220. DOI: 10.1016/j.bpa.2019.05.007

[48] Aaslid R, Lindegaard KF, Sorteberg W, Nornes H. Cerebral autoregulation dynamics in humans. Stroke. 1989;**20**:45-52. DOI: 10.1161/01.str.20.1.45

[49] Willie CK, Tzeng YC, Fisher JA, Ainslie PN. Integrative regulation of human brain blood flow. The Journal of Physiology. 2014;**592**:841-859. DOI: 10.1113/jphysiol.2013.268953

[50] Silverman A, Petersen NH. Physiology, cerebral autoregulation. In: StatPearls. Treasure Island, FL: StatPearls Publishing; 2023

[51] Czosnyka M, Miller C. Participants in the international multidisciplinary consensus conference on multimodality monitoring of cerebral autoregulation. Neurocritical Care. 2014;**21**(Suppl. 2):S95-S102. DOI: 10.1007/s12028-014-0046-0

[52] Le Roux P, Menon DK, Citerio G, Vespa P, Bader MK, Brophy GM, et al. Consensus summary statement of the international multidisciplinary consensus conference on multimodality monitoring in neurocritical care: A statement for healthcare professionals from the Neurocritical Care Society and the European Society of Intensive Care Medicine. Neurocritical Care. 2014;**21**(Suppl. 2):S1-S26. DOI: 10.1007/s12028-014-0041-5

[53] Stern Y. The concept of cognitive reserve: A catalyst for research. Journal of Clinical and Experimental Neuropsychology. 2003;**25**:589-593. DOI: 10.1076/jcen.25.5.589.14571

[54] Pettigrew C, Soldan A. Defining cognitive reserve and implications for cognitive aging. Current Neurology and Neuroscience Reports. 2019;**19**:1. DOI: 10.1007/s11910-019-0917-z

[55] Hoenig MC, Bischof GN, Hammes J, Faber J, Fliessbach K, van Eimeren T, et al. Tau pathology and cognitive reserve in Alzheimer's disease. Neurobiology of Aging. 2017;**57**:1-7. DOI: 10.1016/j.neurobiolaging.2017.05.004

[56] BoylePA, YuL, WilsonRS, LeurgansSE, Schneider JA, Bennett DA. Person-specific contribution of neuropathologies to cognitive loss in old age. Annals of Neurology. 2018;**83**:74-83. DOI: 10.1002/ana.25123

[57] Stern Y. Cognitive reserve. Neuropsychologia. 2009;**47**:2015-2028. DOI: 10.1016/j.neuropsychologia.2009.03.004

[58] Soldan A, Pettigrew C, Albert M. Evaluating cognitive reserve through the prism of preclinical Alzheimer disease. The Psychiatric Clinics of North America. 2018;**41**:65-77. DOI: 10.1016/j.psc.2017.10.006

[59] Cadar D, Lassale C, Davies H, Llewellyn DJ, Batty GD, Steptoe A. Individual and area-based socioeconomic factors associated with dementia incidence in England: Evidence from a 12-year follow-up in the English longitudinal study of ageing. JAMA Psychiatry. 2018;**75**:723-732. DOI: 10.1001/jamapsychiatry.2018.1012

[60] Mosing MA, Lundholm C, Cnattingius S, Gatz M, Pedersen NL. Associations between birth characteristics and age-related cognitive impairment and dementia: A registry-based cohort study. PLoS Medicine. 2018;**15**:e1002609. DOI: 10.1371/journal.pmed.1002609

[61] Stern Y, Arenaza-Urquijo EM, Bartres-Faz D, Belleville S, Cantilon M, Chetelat G, et al. Whitepaper: Defining and investigating cognitive reserve, brain reserve, and brain maintenance. Alzheimer's & Dementia. 2020;**16**:1305-1311. DOI: 10.1016/j.jalz.2018.07.219

[62] Cabeza R, Albert M, Belleville S, Craik FIM, Duarte A, Grady CL, et al. Maintenance, reserve and compensation: The cognitive neuroscience of healthy ageing. Nature Reviews. Neuroscience. 2018;**19**:701-710. DOI: 10.1038/s41583-018-0068-2

[63] Wolf PA. Contributions of the Framingham Heart Study to stroke and dementia epidemiologic research at 60 years. Archives of Neurology. 2012;**69**:567-571. DOI: 10.1001/archneurol.2011.977

[64] Monk TG, Weldon BC, Garvan CW, Dede DE, van der Aa MT, Heilman KM, et al. Predictors of cognitive dysfunction after major noncardiac surgery. Anesthesiology. 2008;**108**:18-30. DOI: 10.1097/01.anes.0000296071.19434.1e

[65] Royse CF, Newman S, Chung F, Stygall J, McKay RE, Boldt J, et al. Development and feasibility of a scale to assess postoperative recovery: The post-operative quality recovery scale. Anesthesiology. 2010;**113**:892-905. DOI: 10.1097/ALN.0b013e3181d960a9

[66] Royse CF, Newman S, Williams Z, Wilkinson DJ. A human volunteer study to identify variability in performance in the cognitive domain of the postoperative quality of recovery scale. Anesthesiology. 2013;**119**:576-581. DOI: 10.1097/ALN.0b013e318299f72b

[67] Bowyer AJ, Heiberg J, Sessler DI, Newman S, Royse AG, Royse CF. Validation of the cognitive recovery assessments

with the Postoperative Quality of Recovery Scale in patients with low-baseline cognition. Anaesthesia. 2018;**73**:1382-1391. DOI: 10.1111/anae.14402

[68] Poitras S, Wood KS, Savard J, Dervin GF, Beaule PE. Assessing functional recovery shortly after knee or hip arthroplasty: A comparison of the clinimetric properties of four tools. BMC Musculoskeletal Disorders. 2016;**17**:478. DOI: 10.1186/s12891-016-1338-7

[69] Sakurai R, Kim Y, Inagaki H, Tokumaru AM, Sakurai K, Shimoji K, et al. MMSE cutoff discriminates hippocampal atrophy: Neural evidence for the cutoff of 24 points. Journal of the American Geriatrics Society. 2021;**69**:839-841. DOI: 10.1111/jgs.17010

[70] Jia X, Wang Z, Huang F, Su C, Du W, Jiang H, et al. A comparison of the Mini-Mental State Examination (MMSE) with the Montreal Cognitive Assessment (MoCA) for mild cognitive impairment screening in Chinese middle-aged and older population: A cross-sectional study. BMC Psychiatry. 2021;**21**:485. DOI: 10.1186/s12888-021-03495-6

[71] Sclan SG, Reisberg B. Functional assessment staging (FAST) in Alzheimer's disease: Reliability, validity, and ordinality. International Psychogeriatrics. 1992;**4**(Suppl. 1):55-69. DOI: 10.1017/s1041610292001157

[72] Na HR, Kim SY, Chang YH, Park MH, Cho ST, Han IW, et al. Functional assessment staging (FAST) in Korean patients with Alzheimer's disease. Journal of Alzheimer's Disease. 2010;**22**:151-158. DOI: 10.3233/JAD-2010-100072

[73] Tan JP, Wang X, Lan X, Li N, Zhang S, Zhao Y, et al. The Epoch effect on cognitive function requires regular updating of cognitive screening tests. Journal of Alzheimer's Disease. 2020;**77**:667-674. DOI: 10.3233/JAD-200112

[74] Schmidt R, Seiler S, Loitfelder M. Longitudinal change of small-vessel disease-related brain abnormalities. Journal of Cerebral Blood Flow & Metabolism. 2016;**36**:26-39. DOI: 10.1038/jcbfm.2015.72

[75] Price CC, Tanner JJ, Schmalfuss I, Garvan CW, Gearen P, Dickey D, et al. A pilot study evaluating presurgery neuroanatomical biomarkers for postoperative cognitive decline after total knee arthroplasty in older adults. Anesthesiology. 2014;**120**:601-613. DOI: 10.1097/ALN.0000000000000080

[76] Meoded A, Huisman T. Diffusion tensor imaging of brain malformations: Exploring the internal architecture. Neuroimaging Clinics of North America. 2019;**29**:423-434. DOI: 10.1016/j.nic.2019.03.004

[77] Lorenz MW, von Kegler S, Steinmetz H, Markus HS, Sitzer M. Carotid intima-media thickening indicates a higher vascular risk across a wide age range: Prospective data from the Carotid Atherosclerosis Progression Study (CAPS). Stroke. 2006;**37**:87-92. DOI: 10.1161/01.STR.0000196964.24024.ea

[78] Purkayastha S, Sorond F. Transcranial Doppler ultrasound: Technique and application. Seminars in Neurology. 2012;**32**:411-420. DOI: 10.1055/s-0032-1331812

[79] Tegeler CH, Crutchfield K, Katsnelson M, Kim J, Tang R, Passmore Griffin L, et al. Transcranial Doppler velocities in a large, healthy population. Journal of Neuroimaging. 2013;**23**:466-472. DOI: 10.1111/j.1552-6569.2012.00711.x

[80] Russell D, Brucher R. Online automatic discrimination between solid and gaseous cerebral microemboli with the first multifrequency transcranial Doppler. Stroke. 2002;**33**:1975-1980. DOI: 10.1161/01.str.0000022809.46400.4b

[81] Martin KK, Wigginton JB, Babikian VL, Pochay VE, Crittenden MD, Rudolph JL. Intraoperative cerebral high-intensity transient signals and postoperative cognitive function: A systematic review. American Journal of Surgery. 2009;**197**:55-63. DOI: 10.1016/j.amjsurg.2007.12.060

[82] Ghosh A, Elwell C, Smith M. Review article: Cerebral near-infrared spectroscopy in adults: A work in progress. Anesthesia & Analgesia. 2012;**115**:1373-1383. DOI: 10.1213/ANE.0b013e31826dd6a6

[83] Ellerkmann RK, Soehle M, Kreuer S. Brain monitoring revisited: What is it all about? Best Practice & Research: Clinical Anaesthesiology. 2013;**27**:225-233. DOI: 10.1016/j.bpa.2013.06.006

[84] Myles PS, Leslie K, McNeil J, Forbes A, Chan MT. Bispectral index monitoring to prevent awareness during anaesthesia: The B-Aware randomised controlled trial. Lancet. 2004;**363**:1757-1763. DOI: 10.1016/S0140-6736(04)16300-9

[85] Avidan MS, Jacobsohn E, Glick D, Burnside BA, Zhang L, Villafranca A, et al. Prevention of intraoperative awareness in a high-risk surgical population. New England Journal of Medicine. 2011;**365**:591-600. DOI: 10.1056/NEJMoa1100403

[86] Mashour GA, Shanks A, Tremper KK, Kheterpal S, Turner CR, Ramachandran SK, et al. Prevention of intraoperative awareness with explicit recall in an unselected surgical population: A randomized comparative effectiveness trial. Anesthesiology. 2012;**117**:717-725. DOI: 10.1097/ALN.0b013e31826904a6

[87] Bijker JB, Persoon S, Peelen LM, Moons KG, Kalkman CJ, Kappelle LJ, et al. Intraoperative hypotension and perioperative ischemic stroke after general surgery: A nested case-control study. Anesthesiology. 2012;**116**:658-664. DOI: 10.1097/ALN.0b013e3182472320

[88] Gottesman RF, Sherman PM, Grega MA, Yousem DM, Borowicz LM Jr, Selnes OA, et al. Watershed strokes after cardiac surgery: Diagnosis, etiology, and outcome. Stroke. 2006;**37**:2306-2311. DOI: 10.1161/01.STR.0000236024.68020.3a

[89] Bijker JB, van Klei WA, Vergouwe Y, Eleveld DJ, van Wolfswinkel L, Moons KG, et al. Intraoperative hypotension and 1-year mortality after noncardiac surgery. Anesthesiology. 2009;**111**:1217-1226. DOI: 10.1097/ALN.0b013e3181c14930

[90] Michelet D, Arslan O, Hilly J, Mangalsuren N, Brasher C, Grace R, et al. Intraoperative changes in blood pressure associated with cerebral desaturation in infants. Paediatric Anaesthesia. 2015;**25**:681-688. DOI: 10.1111/pan.12671

[91] Willingham MD, Avidan MS. Triple low, double low: It's time to deal Achilles heel a single deadly blow. British Journal of Anaesthesia. 2017;**119**:1-4. DOI: 10.1093/bja/aex132

[92] Casati A, Fanelli G, Pietropaoli P, Proietti R, Tufano R, Danelli G, et al. Continuous monitoring of cerebral oxygen saturation in elderly patients undergoing major abdominal surgery minimizes brain exposure to potential hypoxia. Anesthesia and Analgesia.

2005;**101**:740-747. DOI: 10.1213/01.ane.0000166974.96219.cd

[93] Casati A, Fanelli G, Pietropaoli P, Proietti R, Tufano R, Montanini S, et al. Monitoring cerebral oxygen saturation in elderly patients undergoing general abdominal surgery: A prospective cohort study. European Journal of Anaesthesiology. 2007;**24**:59-65. DOI: 10.1017/S0265021506001025

[94] Sessler DI, Sigl JC, Kelley SD, Chamoun NG, Manberg PJ, Saager L, et al. Hospital stay and mortality are increased in patients having a "triple low" of low blood pressure, low bispectral index, and low minimum alveolar concentration of volatile anesthesia. Anesthesiology. 2012;**116**:1195-1203. DOI: 10.1097/ALN.0b013e31825683dc

[95] Kertai MD, Pal N, Palanca BJ, Lin N, Searleman SA, Zhang L, et al. Association of perioperative risk factors and cumulative duration of low bispectral index with intermediate-term mortality after cardiac surgery in the B-Unaware Trial. Anesthesiology. 2010;**112**:1116-1127. DOI: 10.1097/ALN.0b013e3181d5e0a3

[96] Goodman SN, Fanelli D, Ioannidis JP. What does research reproducibility mean? Science Translational Medicine. 2016;**8**:341ps12. DOI: 10.1126/scitranslmed.aaf5027

[97] Whitlock EL, Villafranca AJ, Lin N, Palanca BJ, Jacobsohn E, Finkel KJ, et al. Relationship between bispectral index values and volatile anesthetic concentrations during the maintenance phase of anesthesia in the B-unaware trial. Anesthesiology. 2011;**115**:1209-1218. DOI: 10.1097/ALN.0b013e3182395dcb

[98] Schuller PJ, Newell S, Strickland PA, Barry JJ. Response of bispectral index to neuromuscular block in awake volunteers. British Journal of Anaesthesia. 2015;**115**(Suppl. 1):i95-i103. DOI: 10.1093/bja/aev072

[99] Sessler DI, Turan A, Stapelfeldt WH, Mascha EJ, Yang D, Farag E, et al. Triple-low alerts do not reduce mortality: A real-time randomized trial. Anesthesiology. 2019;**130**:72-82. DOI: 10.1097/ALN.0000000000002480

[100] Georgopoulos AP, James LM, Christova P, Engdahl BE. A two-hit model of the biological origin of posttraumatic stress disorder (PTSD). Journal of Mental health and Clinical Psychology. 2018;**2**:9-14

Chapter 8

Perioperative Preparation of Emergency Patients from Emergency Department to Operating Room

Hany A. Zaki, Eman E. Shaban, Ahmed Shaban,
Baha Hamdi Alkahlout, Nabil A. Shallik
and Aftab Mohammad Azad

Abstract

Perioperative preparation for emergency patients is paramount, as it entails a comprehensive approach to ensure the safety, well-being, and successful outcomes of individuals facing urgent surgical interventions. In the preoperative phase, rapid but essential steps are taken, such as assessing the patient's medical history, conducting diagnostic tests, and stabilising their condition to minimise risks during surgery. So in this chapter, we will discuss the importance of formation of the multidisciplinary team, efficiency improvements, identifying the need for emergency department (ED) to operating room (OR) Handoff Standardisation, and integration of ED nurses into the OR. It begins by establishing the criteria for identifying patients needing urgent surgery, encompassing traumatic injuries and acute medical conditions. It extensively covers the interdisciplinary collaboration required among ED staff, OR teams, anaesthesiologists, surgeons, and nurses. The scope includes patient assessment and stabilisation procedures conducted in the ED, focusing on diagnostics, interventions, and life-saving measures. Furthermore, the chapter delves into handoff protocols and communication strategies, highlighting their crucial role in ensuring safe and efficient patient transfers. It addresses resource allocation, emphasising the optimisation of operating rooms, equipment, and personnel. The chapter also acknowledges the importance of patient and family engagement, stressing clear communication, informed consent, and emotional support.

Keywords: perioperative preparation, emergency patients, emergency room, operating room, emergency department

1. Introduction

1.1 Perioperative care

Perioperative care, as defined in the discussion, is a comprehensive system of medical strategies to ensure patient well-being throughout the surgical journey [1]. It comprises three essential phases: preoperative, intraoperative, and postoperative care.

In the preoperative phase, healthcare professionals meticulously prepare patients for surgery through assessments such as blood tests, scans, and psychological counselling, ensuring they are physically and mentally ready for the procedure. During the volatile intraoperative phase, nurses and anaesthesiologists monitor vital signs, maintain a sterile environment, and prioritise safety in the operating room. Postoperative care focuses on patient recovery, including pain management, wound care, and monitoring progress in the Post Anaesthesia Care Unit (PACU) [2]. Comprehensive perioperative care is vital as it not only enhances the patient experience by alleviating stress but also contributes to better health outcomes, enabling patients to return to normal life faster and reducing healthcare costs per capita. Integrating digital health solutions, such as the Buddy Care Platform, further streamlines and enhances perioperative care by facilitating remote monitoring, patient engagement, and data collection, ultimately making healthcare more accessible and patient-centred [2]. Essentially, perioperative care encompasses a holistic approach to surgical patients' well-being, from preparation to recovery, focusing on safety, comfort, and efficient healthcare delivery.

1.2 Importance of perioperative preparation for emergency patients

Perioperative preparation for emergency patients is paramount, as it entails a comprehensive approach to ensure the safety, well-being, and successful outcomes of individuals facing urgent surgical interventions. In these critical moments, when time is of the essence, the significance of perioperative care pathways becomes evident. These preoperative, intraoperative, and postoperative phases offer a structured framework for healthcare professionals to navigate the complexities of emergency surgeries. In the preoperative phase, rapid but essential steps are taken, such as assessing the patient's medical history, conducting diagnostic tests, and stabilising their condition to minimise risks during surgery. The surgical team takes centre stage in the intraoperative stage, meticulously monitoring vital signs, maintaining sterile conditions, and responding swiftly to unforeseen challenges that may arise, especially in emergencies involving life-threatening conditions such as trauma or ruptured organs. While shorter in emergency cases, postoperative care is equally critical, involving continuous monitoring, pain management, and vigilance against complications, ensuring a smooth recovery process.

Beyond the immediate medical aspects, perioperative care pathways also prioritise the patient experience, recognising emergency situations' emotional and psychological tolls. Compassionate and comprehensive care reduces patient anxiety and enhances their satisfaction with the healthcare system. Moreover, efficient perioperative care pathways contribute to cost-effectiveness by optimising resource allocation, minimising hospital stays, and preventing complications. With the rising demand for surgical interventions, particularly in emergencies, these pathways help healthcare systems meet the challenges of an evolving healthcare landscape. Central to perioperative care is collaboration among healthcare professionals, including surgeons, anaesthesiologists, nurses, and specialists, fostering an interdisciplinary approach that enhances patient safety and care quality. In essence, perioperative preparation for emergency patients is a holistic endeavour, ensuring that individuals receive the best possible care during critical junctures in their healthcare journey, where timely, effective, and compassionate care can make all the difference in their outcomes and overall well-being (**Figure 1**).

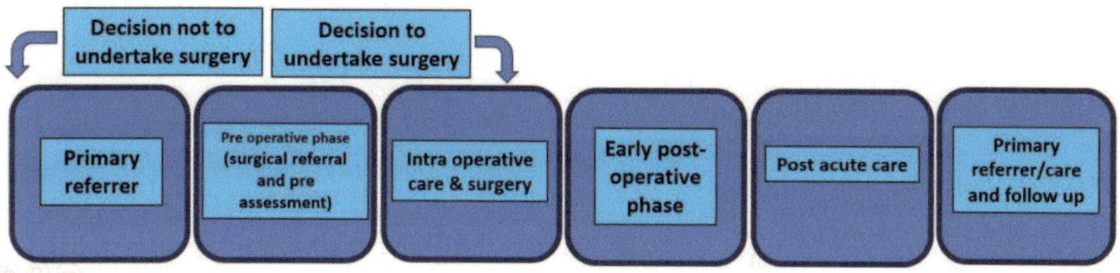

Figure 1.
Perioperative care journey. Source [2].

1.3 Overview of the transition from the emergency department (ED) to the operating room (OR)

According to Atzema and Maclagan [3], the transition from the emergency department (ED) to the operating room (OR) involves a standardised handoff process that was developed by a multidisciplinary team to improve patient care and efficiency. This process was motivated by the success of similar handoff processes in other departments, such as from the OR to PICU and NICU to the OR. Here is an overview of the transition from the ED to the OR:

1.3.1 Formation of the multidisciplinary team

The journey to standardise the transition from the emergency department (ED) to the operating room (OR) began with the formation of a multidisciplinary team. An adverse event did not prompt this initiative but rather the success of standardising handoff processes in other hospital departments [3]. The team comprised frontline staff from various departments, including Respiratory Therapy, ICU Nursing, OR Nursing, Anaesthesiology, and Paediatric Intensivists. The motivation behind this collaboration was to establish a more structured and intentional transition of care for patients moving from the ED to the OR.

The team did not anticipate the level of efficiency the new handoff process would bring. Anaesthesiology teams could transport patients to the Paediatric Intensive Care Unit (PICU) significantly faster than before. This initiative also encouraged staff to ask more pertinent questions during handoffs and created an environment where parents could observe the process without hesitation. These initial successes fuelled the team's determination to continue improving the handoff process. Also, it is crucial to include the emergency drugs in "Critical Medication Bag" including basic ACLS medicines for all critical patient transports for the management of any emergency scenarios.

1.3.2 Efficiency improvements

One of the remarkable outcomes of the new handoff process was the substantial improvement in efficiency. For example, the Anaesthesiology teams saw a 25% reduction in the time it took to transfer patients to the PICU. Similarly, in the Neonatal Intensive Care Unit (NICU), report times decreased from an average of 16 minutes to just 6 minutes, even when including the transfer of the baby from the cart to the bed [3]. These improvements directly resulted from enhanced communication and a more streamlined handoff process that became integral to daily healthcare routines.

The success of this transition process was built on the idea that when all stakeholders in patient care are involved in the process improvement efforts, the results can be exceptional. The team's collaboration involved six different departments and seven distinct roles, emphasising the importance of each component in delivering efficient and safe patient care. As the handoff process continued to evolve and improve, ongoing engagement with staff from the Emergency Department, OR, and Anaesthesiology was crucial to maintaining these positive outcomes. The experience revealed that the best solutions often emerge when those directly involved in patient care come together, making the standardisation of the ED-to-OR handoff a prime example of healthcare improvement [4].

1.3.3 Identifying the need for ED to OR handoff standardisation

While standardisation of handoff processes existed in various healthcare settings, the transition of patients from the emergency department (ED) to the operating room (OR) had yet to be thoroughly addressed [4]. This was a critical gap in patient care, especially for Class A surgeries that required swift and efficient transfers. The relationship between the ED and the OR was often strained due to the urgency of these cases, which further underscored the need for a standardised process.

1.3.4 Identifying key roles

While developing the standardised handoff, the team recognised that the ED nurse often possessed the most comprehensive information about the patient, including vital situational awareness. This information was highly relevant to Anaesthesiology and OR Nursing, as it impacted their ability to provide timely and appropriate care to the patient [4]. Realising that the ED nurse played a pivotal role in the handoff process was a crucial insight that guided the subsequent improvements.

1.3.5 Integration of ED nurses into the OR

The team decided that the ED nurse and the Surgical Resident would accompany the patient directly to the assigned OR room to facilitate a seamless handoff process, especially in emergencies. This proactive approach ensured the ED nurse could provide essential information and context during the handoff. It was a practical solution that eliminated ambiguity about whether ED nurses were welcome in the OR, a concern that had previously hindered efficient handoffs. Additionally, the minimal requirement for the ED nurse to don a surgical mask and hat streamlined the transition further.

1.3.6 Importance of full attention during handoff

Recognising the importance of focused attention during the handoff, the team scripted specific steps to ensure effective communication. The Surgical Resident would announce critical patient details and procedures upon entering the OR room. Anaesthesiology would call for a moment of quiet, and the ED nurse would deliver a report tailored to the severity of the patient's condition. This scripting provided clarity and emphasised the need for everyone involved to actively engage and concentrate on the handoff.

1.3.7 Continued collaboration

The success of the transition from the ED to the OR was a testament to the power of collaboration among various departments and roles within the hospital. This complex process involved six departments and seven distinct roles, all essential to its improvement. These groups' ongoing collaboration and engagement were crucial for the continued success and sustainability of the standardised handoff process [4]. The experience underscored the principle that those closest to work often have the best insights into solving the associated problems, making this process a shining example of healthcare improvement through teamwork and communication.

1.4 Purpose and scope of the chapter

The chapter on "Perioperative Preparation of Emergency Patients from ED to OR" serves a critical purpose by exploring the intricacies of transitioning emergency patients from the ED to the OR. Its primary objective is to enhance the clinical understanding of healthcare professionals, equipping them with the knowledge and skills necessary to navigate the unique challenges presented by critically ill patients requiring surgical intervention following emergencies. This chapter prioritises patient safety and resource efficiency, emphasising the importance of standardised protocols for information exchange, equipment readiness, and interdisciplinary collaboration. It begins by establishing the criteria for identifying patients needing urgent surgery, encompassing traumatic injuries and acute medical conditions. It extensively covers the interdisciplinary collaboration required among ED staff, OR teams, anaesthesiologists, surgeons, and nurses. The scope includes patient assessment and stabilisation procedures conducted in the ED, focusing on diagnostics, interventions, and life-saving measures.

Furthermore, the chapter delves into handoff protocols and communication strategies, highlighting their crucial role in ensuring safe and efficient patient transfers. It addresses resource allocation, emphasising the optimisation of operating rooms, equipment, and personnel. The chapter also acknowledges the importance of patient and family engagement, stressing clear communication, informed consent, and emotional support.

2. The role of the emergency department in patient evaluation and stabilisation

2.1 Initial assessment and triage in the ED

Initial assessment and triage in the ED are a critical process that is pivotal in providing timely and appropriate care to patients, especially in paediatric cases. The Paediatric Assessment Triangle (PAT) is a valuable tool for rapidly and systematically evaluating a child's condition upon arrival at the ED [5]. The first step in triage involves a quick assessment of appearance, breathing, and circulation (ABC) using PAT. This initial visual and auditory assessment helps categorise the patient's illness as stable or unstable. Unstable conditions are further classified into life-threatening and non-life threatening. Patients in the former category, such as those with cardiac arrest, cardio-respiratory failure, decompensated shock, deep coma, or severe stridor, require immediate resuscitation (**Figure 2**).

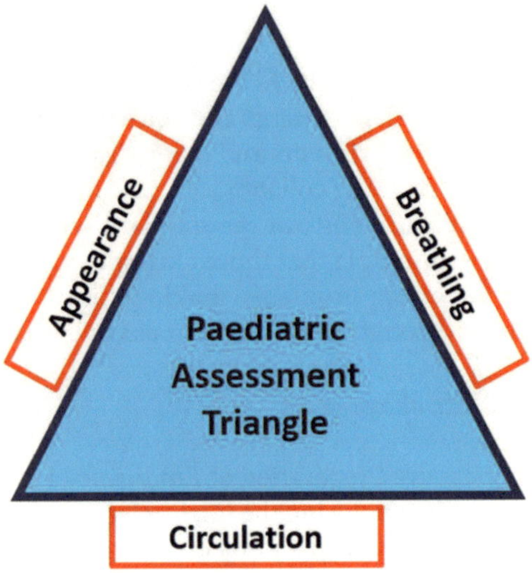

Figure 2.
Paediatric assessment triangle (PAT) (source: [5]).

Once a child is on the path to stabilisation, the primary assessment (ABCDE approach) is conducted. This involves a detailed examination of the airway (A), breathing (B), circulation (C), neurologic abnormalities (D), and a head-to-toe examination (Exposure). This thorough assessment, completed within 1–3 minutes, helps determine the patient's physiological abnormalities and assigns them to one of five levels of acuity: Resuscitation, Emergent care, Urgent care, Less urgent, or Non-urgent care [5].

The goals of the triage system in the ED are to ensure that the right patient receives the right care from the right provider at the right time to achieve the right outcome. This involves rapidly identifying patients with life-threatening illnesses, initiating appropriate first-aid measures, and continuously monitoring paediatric patients who can deteriorate rapidly. The general PAT assessment is crucial in identifying patients requiring immediate life-saving interventions. Appearance, work of breathing, and circulation are assessed to determine the child's condition. Abnormal findings in any of these categories may indicate a need for urgent attention.

2.2 Diagnostic procedures in the ED

Advancements in medical technology over the last 25 years have revolutionised emergency medicine, particularly in diagnostic procedures. EDs faced limitations in obtaining diagnostic information in the past, relying mainly on basic lab tests and plain radiographs [6]. However, the landscape has shifted dramatically with the advent of cutting-edge diagnostic tools and improved accessibility to these tests. Today, the emergency department serves as a hub for diagnostic testing, where physicians can efficiently coordinate a patient's care, and most test results are available within a few hours. This rapid turnaround time is critical in initiating prompt and definitive care, significantly impacting patient outcomes. Advanced diagnostic imaging modalities such as ultrasounds, CT scans, and even MRI studies can be obtained swiftly, allowing for timely diagnoses of conditions such as intracranial haemorrhage, pulmonary embolism, aortic aneurysm, and more [7].

Nevertheless, the ease of obtaining these diagnostic studies comes at a cost. The American College of Radiology reports that diagnostic imaging is the fastest growing medical expenditure in the United States, with an annual growth rate of 9%, triple that of general medical expenditures [6]. Over the past decade, the number of MRI and CT scans performed in EDs quadrupled, and ultrasounds more than doubled. Despite these technological advances, it is crucial to emphasise that diagnostic testing should differ from the importance of a thorough history and physical examination (H&PE) [8]. Before ordering any diagnostic test, clinicians should consider several key questions. They should contemplate how the test results will guide their actions, whether the test will help confirm or exclude a diagnosis, and how the results will impact their overall diagnostic strategy, management plan, or final decision regarding patient disposition. These questions are valuable guides when deciding whether to order a diagnostic test, whether a simple blood test or a costly imaging study.

It is important to note that diagnostic tests should primarily aim to rule in or rule out specific conditions based on the patient's presenting symptoms and the differential diagnosis generated from their H&PE [7]. However, tests are often ordered for various reasons, including clinical suspicion, established practices, perceived standard of care, requests from consultants or primary care physicians, patient requests, and risk management considerations. Sometimes, diagnostic workups may be influenced by pattern recognition and anecdotal experience, highlighting the blend of art and science in medicine. Consultant physicians can also influence the choice of diagnostic tests [6]. For instance, when a patient presents with abdominal pain, a consultant may request specific tests. However, normal test results should not sway the clinician's clinical suspicion, and it is an opportunity to educate colleagues about the utility of certain tests in specific contexts.

Statistical considerations play a crucial role in understanding diagnostic testing. Sensitivity and specificity are fundamental concepts. Sensitivity refers to the likelihood of a test being positive in the presence of a disease. At the same time, specificity pertains to the likelihood of a negative test without disease. Tests with high sensitivity are effective at ruling out disease, whereas those with high specificity are good at ruling it in. Positive and negative predictive values (PPV and NPV) consider the prevalence of disease in the population and influence the reliability of a test result [7]. Communication with patients about the rationale behind test orders is essential to manage expectations.

The concept of pretest and post-test probability is also valuable in evaluating the significance of diagnostic test results. It involves considering the patient's risk factors, clinical presentation, and test outcomes. While evidence-based guidelines exist for many conditions, medicine encompasses science and art, and there may be times when a particular test is not indicated. Bedside ultrasound by emergency physicians has become increasingly prevalent in recent years [6]. This technology allows for rapid assessments and has been shown to improve patient outcomes and the efficiency of care in the ED. It aids in making decisions regarding speciality consultations, operative management, and patient dispositions, often reducing the time needed for these critical determinations.

2.3 Communication between ED and OR teams

Effective communication between the ED and OR teams is paramount in ensuring patient safety and seamless care transitions, particularly in high-stress situations where quick decisions and rapid responses are essential. The significance of communication in healthcare settings, including the ED, has been underscored by various studies, acknowledging that patient safety incidents often occur due to communication breakdowns. A study published in The Journal of Emergency Medicine highlighted the critical role of communication in the ED and its implications for patient care excellence [9]. The authors found that poor ED communication contributed significantly to unfortunate patient outcomes. One prominent issue was inadequate and ineffective staff communication, a challenge exacerbated within the demanding environment of the ED. Problems with the transfer of medical information and orders, especially during shift handoffs, were identified as communication-based factors impacting patient safety. Instances where changes in vital signs were not promptly communicated to attending physicians led to patient safety incidents. Delays in treatment due to communication failures were documented, illustrating the dire consequences of inadequate communication within the ED [9].

Medication management issues, such as incorrect doses, medication errors, delays, and miscalculations, were also attributed to communication problems within the ED. Compliance with patient safety protocols, such as infection control, proper clerical and laboratory processes, and complete discharge instructions, was emphasised as areas where communication lapses could compromise patient safety [10]. Strategies for improving ED outcomes have been proposed to address these communication challenges. One key issue is ambient noise within the ED, which can hinder effective communication. Solutions include noise monitoring, equipment alarm adjustments, and using single-person rooms to reduce noise levels. Communication schemes, such as urgency-based plans and limited overhead paging, have effectively enhanced communication efficiency [10]. Recognising that different healthcare roles require tailored communication approaches and acknowledging the varying communication needs of physicians, nurses, and staff can improve information transfer.

Attention to team dynamics is also crucial. Provider organisations with strong teamwork and communication principles deliver higher-quality care while reducing costs. The Joint Commission has identified communication failures as a common cause of sentinel events. Therefore, promoting teamwork and effective communication within the ED is essential [10]. Implementing daily interdisciplinary huddles, establishing communication channels for departmental information sharing, and encouraging feedback from frontline staff can enhance communication and foster a culture of continuous improvement.

3. Preoperative assessment and planning

3.1 Transfer of care from ED to surgical team

A patient transitioning from the Emergency Department to the surgical team marks the crucial starting point of preoperative assessment and planning. This transition is the foundation for ensuring the patient's safety and well-being throughout the surgical process. It involves establishing a solid partnership between the anaesthesiologist and the patient. This partnership is built upon mutual understanding, which involves outlining the anaesthesia technique and recognising any associated risks. Simultaneously, it aims to offer premedication drugs and carry out necessary interventions before surgery [11]. A key aspect of risk assessment involves tailored investigations and referrals from other medical specialities. Effective preoperative assessment helps prevent last-minute delays or postponements of surgery, ensuring a smoother and more efficient process.

3.2 Comprehensive patient evaluation

A thorough preoperative evaluation is the cornerstone of optimal surgical preparation. It encompasses a detailed patient history, comprehensive physical examination, and essential laboratory investigations. The history-taking process delves into past adverse reactions to anaesthesia, difficulties with intravenous access, airway management complications, extended recovery times, postoperative nausea and vomiting, and delirium experiences. It also considers specific details, such as whether the patient is scheduled for elective or emergency surgery, if they have cardiac issues undergoing non-cardiac procedures, or if they are taking anticoagulants, among other factors [12]. Assessing functional status through comprehensive measures is crucial for geriatric patients to identify those at risk and anticipate potential complications. This comprehensive evaluation includes recording all medications, doses, and a detailed history of over-the-counter and herbal drugs, illicit substance use, addiction history, malignant hyperthermia susceptibility, and other adverse reactions [11]. Anthropometric measurements and hemodynamic parameters should also be documented. The examination must carefully inspect the airway and spine and systematically review various organ systems, ensuring a holistic understanding of the patient's health.

3.3 Identifying comorbidities and special considerations

The healthcare landscape has evolved over the years, resulting in many surgical candidates with advanced age and multiple comorbidities, often on multiple medications. This shift has necessitated adaptations in perioperative patient care. Identifying comorbidities and addressing special considerations are critical steps in preoperative planning. Risk assessment tools, such as the American Society of Anaesthesiologists physical status (ASA PS) grading, aid in shaping the anaesthesia plan. However, while valuable, these tools may only encompass some preoperative physiological and functional aspects, the type of surgery, and postoperative care [13]. To enhance comorbidity assessment, age-adjusted scores, such as the National Surgical Quality Improvement Programme (NSQIP) model, the Charlson comorbidity index (CCI), or the revised cardiac risk index (RCRI), are recommended, particularly for cardiac perioperative risk stratification. Functional status, often measured in metabolic equivalents (METS), quantifies an individual's exercise capacity and ability to withstand surgical stress. Cardiopulmonary exercise testing (CPET) provides a more in-depth assessment but requires specialised facilities and trained personnel [12]. Surgical risk varies based on the type of procedure, with minor surgeries presenting lower cardiovascular risk and major surgeries, such as peripheral vascular or transplant surgeries, associated with higher-risk percentages.

3.4 Informed consent and shared decision-making

Preoperative assessment tools must align with patient sensitivities in an era of heightened patient awareness, knowledge, and safety expectations. Informed consent and shared decision-making have taken on greater significance. Patients should be informed about the planned surgery, potential risks, and alternative options. Engaging patients in these discussions empowers them to actively participate in their care journey [12]. Additionally, when evaluating patients for surgery, special attention should be given to identifying risk factors related to obstructive sleep apnoea (OSA).

Although polysomnography is the gold standard for diagnosing OSA, its routine use as a screening tool is impractical [11]. Various questionnaires, such as the STOP-Bang questionnaire, can aid in identifying patients at risk for OSA. These assessments help tailor perioperative care plans to mitigate OSA-related complications. Preoperative investigations should be guided by protocols, such as those outlined by the Indian Society of Anaesthesiologists, taking into account the patient's circumstances and validity periods of previous tests [14].

3.5 Preoperative optimisation/prehabilitation

Preparing patients for surgery involves assessing risks and optimising their physical condition. Preoperative optimisation minimises perioperative complications, such as bronchospasm, aspiration, pulmonary infections, wound infections, and myocardial events [11]. Optimisation strategies may include lifestyle modifications such as smoking and alcohol cessation, adjustments to antihypertensive and antidiabetic treatments, incentive spirometry to improve lung function, management of anaemia, and enhancement of exercise tolerance [12]. Prehabilitation, a related concept, focuses on improving physical functionality through exercises tailored to specific surgical procedures. While direct evidence of its impact on postoperative pain and functionality remains under investigation, prehabilitation has shown promise in reducing rehabilitation unit admissions. Emotional and psychological support through preoperative counselling also helps alleviate patient anxiety and fear, enhancing their overall surgical experience [15].

3.6 Decision to defer surgery

Finally, the decision to defer surgery is a patient-specific assessment that considers factors such as medication use, the severity of comorbidities, surgical risk, and hypertension control. Different types of surgeries have varying thresholds for postponement. Urgency, institutional practices, monitoring capabilities, and clinician and patient preferences all influence this decision. High-risk procedures, especially those impacting airway or cardiopulmonary function, may necessitate a lower threshold for surgery delay, particularly for patients with uncontrolled obstructive sleep apnoea (OSA) [11, 16]. Preoperative evaluation clinics play a vital role in making these determinations, along with the availability of sleep testing when needed.

Author details

Hany A. Zaki[1], Eman E. Shaban[2], Ahmed Shaban[3], Baha Hamdi Alkahlout[1,4,5], Nabil A. Shallik[6,7,8]* and Aftab Mohammad Azad[1,5]

1 Emergency Medicine, Hamad Medical Corporation, Doha, Qatar

2 Al Jufairi Diagnosis and Treatment, MOH, Doha, Qatar

3 Internal Medicine - Mansoura General Hospital, Egypt

4 Emergency Medicine, Weill Cornell Medical College in Qatar, Doha, Qatar

5 Emergency Medicine, College of Medicine, Qatar University, Doha, Qatar

6 Anaesthesia, ICU and Perioperative Medicine, Hamad Medical Corporation, Doha, Qatar

7 Clinical Anesthesiology, Weill Cornell Medical College in Qatar, Doha, Qatar

8 Clinical Anesthesiology, Qatar University, Doha, Qatar

*Address all correspondence to: nabilsholik66@hotmail.com

References

[1] Karioja P. What is Perioperative Care? [Online]. 2021. Available from: https://www.buddyhealthcare.com/en/blog/what-is-perioperative-care; www.buddyhealthcare.com

[2] CPOC. What is Perioperative Care? Centre for Perioperative Care [Online]. 2023. Available from: https://cpoc.org.uk/about-cpoc/what-perioperative-care; cpoc.org.uk

[3] Atzema CL, Maclagan LC. The transition of care between emergency department and primary care: A scoping study. Academic Emergency Medicine. 2017;**24**(2):201-215. DOI: 10.1111/acem.13125

[4] Medcom. Standardizing Emergency Department to Operating Room handoff for Class A surgery - The Loop [Online] The Loop. 2015. Available from: https://medcom.uiowa.edu/theloop/quest-newsletter/standardizing-emergency-department-to-operating-room-handoff-for-class-a-surgery

[5] Jayashree M, Singhi SC. Initial assessment and triage in ER. The Indian Journal of Pediatrics. 2011;**78**(9):1100-1108. DOI: 10.1007/s12098-011-0411-3

[6] SAEM. Diagnostic Testing in the Emergency Department Default [Online]. 2022. Available from: https://www.saem.org/about-saem/academies-interest-groups-affiliates2/cdem/for-students/online-education/m3-curriculum/group-diagnostic-testing/diagnostic-testing-in-the-emergency-department

[7] Kayathri P. What Are the Diagnostic Tests Done in an Emergency Setup? [Online]. 2023. Available from: https://www.icliniq.com/articles/first-aid-and-emergencies/diagnostic-tests-during-emergency; www.icliniq.com [Accessed: September 4, 2023]

[8] Shallik N, Zaghw A, Dogan Z, Rahman W. The use of virtual endoscopy for diagnosis of traumatic supra-glottic airway stenosis. JCAO. 2017;**2**(103):2

[9] Healthline. Improving Communication in the Emergency Room Default [online]. 2021. Available from: https://www.healthstream.com/resource/blog/improving-communication-in-the-emergency-room

[10] O'Daniel M, Rosenstein AH. Professional Communication and Team Collaboration NCBI [Online]. 2018. Available from: https://www.ncbi.nlm.nih.gov/books/NBK2637/

[11] Jindal P, Patil V, Pradhan R, Mahajan HC, Rani A, Pabba UG. Update on preoperative evaluation and optimisation. Indian Journal of Anaesthesia [online]. 2023;**67**(1):39-47. DOI: 10.4103/ija.ija_1041_22

[12] Teach Me Surgery. The Pre-Operative Assessment - TeachMeSurgery [online]. TeachMeSurgery. 2018. Available from: https://teachmesurgery.com/perioperative/preoperative/assessment/

[13] Shallik N, Karmakar A. Is it time for high flow nasal oxygen to be included in the difficult airway algorithm? British Journal of Anaesthesia. 2018;**121**(2):511-512

[14] Shallik N. Anesthetic Management for Drug Induced Sleep Endoscopy. Middle East Journal of Anaesthesiology. 2015;**23**(2):131-135

[15] Dardeer A, Shallik N. Perioperative anaphylaxis: A new visit to an old topic.

Trends in Anaesthesia and Critical Care. 2019;**26**(27):1e10

[16] Dardeer A, Alhammad MF, Shallik NA. Anesthesia management in OSA patient. In: Delakorda M, de Vries N. (eds) The Role of Epiglottis in Obstructive Sleep Apnea. Cham: Springer; 2023. DOI: 10.1007/978-3-031-34992-8_26